Updates in Head and Neck Cancer

Editors

SARAH L. ROHDE
EBEN L. ROSENTHAL

SURGICAL ONCOLOGY CLINICS OF NORTH AMERICA

www.surgonc.theclinics.com

Consulting Editor
TIMOTHY M. PAWLIK

October 2024 • Volume 33 • Number 4

ELSEVIER

1600 John F. Kennedy Boulevard • Suite 1800 • Philadelphia, Pennsylvania, 19103-2899

http://www.theclinics.com

SURGICAL ONCOLOGY CLINICS OF NORTH AMERICA Volume 33, Number 4
October 2024 ISSN 1055-3207, ISBN-13: 978-0-443-12961-2

Editor: John Vassallo (j.vassallo@elsevier.com)
Developmental Editor: Malvika Shah

Surgical Oncology Clinics of North America (ISSN 1055-3207) is published quarterly by Elsevier Inc., 360 Park Avenue South, New York, NY 10010-1710. Months of publication are January, April, July, and October. Business and Editorial Offices: 1600 John F. Kennedy Blvd., Ste. 1800, Philadelphia, PA 19103-2899. Customer Service Office: 3251 Riverport Lane, Maryland Heights, MO 63043. Periodicals postage paid at New York, NY and additional mailing offices. Subscription prices are $345.00 per year (US individuals), $100.00 (US student/resident), $385.00 (Canadian individuals), $100.00 (Canadian student/resident), $499.00 (foreign individuals), and $205.00 (foreign student/resident). For institutional access pricing please contact Customer Service via the contact information below. Foreign air speed delivery is included in all *Clinics* subscription prices. All prices are subject to change without notice. Orders, claims, and journal inquiries: Please visit our Support Hub page https://service.elsevier.com for assistance.

Reprints. For copies of 100 or more, of articles in this publication, please contact the Commercial Reprints Department, Elsevier Inc., 360 Park Avenue South, New York, New York 10010-1710. Tel. 212-633-3874; Fax: 212-633-3820; E-mail: reprints@elsevier.com.

Surgical Oncology Clinics of North America is covered in *MEDLINE/PubMed (Index Medicus)* and *EMBASE/ Excerpta Medica, Current Contents/Clinical Medicine,* and *ISI/BIOMED.*

Contributors

CONSULTING EDITOR

TIMOTHY M. PAWLIK, MD, PhD, MPH, MTS, MBA, FACS, FSSO, FRACS (Hon.)
Professor and Chair, Department of Surgery; The Urban Meyer III and Shelley Meyer Chair
for Cancer Research; Professor of Surgery, Oncology, and Health Services Management
and Policy; Surgeon in Chief; The Ohio State University, Wexner Medical Center,
Columbus, Ohio

EDITORS

SARAH L. ROHDE, MD, MMHC
Associate Professor and Chief of Head and Neck Oncologic Surgery, Director,
Department of Otolaryngology–Head and Neck Surgery, Vanderbilt University Medical
Center, Nashville, Tennessee

EBEN L. ROSENTHAL, MD
Barry Baker Professor and Chair, Department of Otolaryngology–Head and Neck Surgery,
Vanderbilt University Medical Center, Nashville, Tennessee

AUTHORS

GABRIELA A. CALCANO, BS
Student, Department of Otolaryngology–Head and Neck Surgery, Mayo Clinic, Rochester,
Minnesota

JOHN CEREMSAK, MD
Surgical Resident, Department of Otolaryngology–Head and Neck Surgery, Vanderbilt
University Medical Center, Nashville, Tennessee

JENNIFER CHOE, MD, PhD
Assistant Professor, Division of Hematology/Oncology, Department of Medicine,
Vanderbilt-Ingram Cancer Center, Vanderbilt University Medical Center, Nashville,
Tennessee

ZAINAB FARZAL, MD, MPH
Fellow, Department of Otolaryngology–Head and Neck Surgery, University of California
San Francisco, San Francisco, California; Department of Otolaryngology–Head and Neck
Surgery, University of Texas Southwestern Medical Center, Dallas, Texas

DANIELLE FISHMAN, MD
Resident Physician, Division of Hematology/Oncology, Department of Medicine,
Vanderbilt-Ingram Cancer Center, Vanderbilt University Medical Center, Nashville,
Tennessee

DANIELLE M. GILLARD, MD
Resident, Department of Otolaryngology–Head and Neck Surgery, University of California
San Francisco, San Francisco, California

EVAN M. GRABOYES, MD, MPH
Associate Professor, Departments of Otolaryngology–Head and Neck Surgery, and Public Health Sciences, Hollings Cancer Center, Medical University of South Carolina, Charleston, South Carolina

GABRIEL A. HERNANDEZ-HERRERA, BS
Student, Department of Otolaryngology–Head and Neck Surgery, Mayo Clinic, Rochester, Minnesota

MELANIE HICKS, MD
Assistant Professor, Department of Otolaryngology–Head and Neck Surgery, Vanderbilt University Medical Center, Nashville, Tennessee

COLLEEN G. HOCHFELDER, MD, MS
Resident Physician, Department of Otolaryngology–Head and Neck Surgery, University of Michigan, Ann Arbor, Michigan

MICHAEL M. LI, MD
Fellow, Department of Otolaryngology–Head and Neck Surgery, The Ohio State University James Cancer Center, Columbus, Ohio

KYLE MANNION, MD
Associate Professor, Department of Otolaryngology–Head and Neck Surgery, Vanderbilt University Medical Center, Nashville, Tennessee

ALEJANDRO R. MARRERO-GONZALEZ, BS
Student, Department of Otolaryngology–Head and Neck Surgery, Medical University of South Carolina, Charleston, South Carolina

LAUREN E. MILLER, MD, MBA
Fellow, Department of Otolaryngology–Head and Neck Surgery, The Ohio State University James Cancer Center, Columbus, Ohio

ALEX A. NAGELSCHNEIDER, MD
Assistant Professor, Department of Radiology, Mayo Clinic, Rochester, Minnesota

MATTHEW OLD, MD
Professor, Department of Otolaryngology–Head and Neck Surgery, The Ohio State University James Cancer Center, Columbus, Ohio

BIREN K. PATEL, MBBS
Post Doctoral Research Fellow, Department of Neurosurgery, Emory University, Atlanta, Georgia

RAMEZ PHILIPS, MD
Instructor, Department of Otolaryngology–Head and Neck Surgery, Vanderbilt University Medical Center, Nashville, Tennessee

GUSTAVO PRADILLA, MD
Professor, Departments of Neurosurgery and Otolaryngology–Head and Neck Surgery, Emory University, Atlanta, Georgia

TAM RAMSEY, MD
Fellow, Department of Otolaryngology–Head and Neck Surgery, University of Cincinnati, College of Medicine, Cincinnati, Ohio

ALEJANDRA RODAS, MD
Post Doctoral Research Fellow, Department of Otolaryngology–Head and Neck Surgery, Emory University, Atlanta, Georgia

DAVID M. ROUTMAN, MD
Assistant Professor, Department of Radiation Oncology, Mayo Clinic, Rochester, Minnesota

WILLIAM R. RYAN, MD
Professor, Department of Otolaryngology–Head and Neck Surgery, University of California San Francisco, San Francisco, California

CECELIA E. SCHMALBACH, MD, MSc
The David Myers, MD Professor and Chair, Department of Otolaryngology–Head and Neck Surgery, Lewis Katz School of Medicine at Temple Hospital, Philadelphia, Pennsylvania

ANDREW G. SHUMAN, MD
Associate Professor, Department of Otolaryngology–Head and Neck Surgery, University of Michigan, Ann Arbor, Michigan

C. ARTURO SOLARES, MD, FACS
Professor, Departments of Otolaryngology–Head and Neck Surgery, and Neurosurgery, Emory University, Atlanta, Georgia

ALICE L. TANG, MD
Associate Professor, Fellowship Director, Department of Otolaryngology–Head and Neck Surgery, University of Cincinnati, College of Medicine, Cincinnati, Cincinnati, Ohio

LEONARDO TARICIOTTI, MD
Post Doctoral Research Fellow, Department of Neurosurgery, Emory University, Atlanta, Georgia

RAISA TIKHTMAN, MD
Resident Physician, Department of Otolaryngology–Head and Neck Surgery, University of Cincinnati College of Medicine, Cincinnati, Ohio

MICHAEL C. TOPF, MD, MSCI
Assistant Professor, Department of Otolaryngology–Head and Neck Surgery, Vanderbilt University Medical Center, Vanderbilt University School of Engineering, Nashville, Tennessee

KATHRYN M. VAN ABEL, MD
Professor, Department of Otolaryngology–Head and Neck Surgery, Mayo Clinic, Rochester, Minnesota

PRATYUSHA YALAMANCHI, MD
Instructor, Department of Otolaryngology–Head and Neck Surgery, Vanderbilt University Medical Center, Nashville, Tennessee

FLORA YAN, MD
Resident, Department of Otolaryngology–Head and Neck Surgery, Lewis Katz School of Medicine at Temple Hospital, Philadelphia, Pennsylvania

WENDA YE, MD
Surgical Resident, Department of Otolaryngology–Head and Neck Surgery, Vanderbilt University Medical Center, Nashville, Tennessee

Contents

The use of immunotherapy in head and neck squamous cell carcinoma (HNSCC)has increased treatment options for patients who may not be candidates for traditional cytotoxic chemotherapy. Recent studies have resulted in the approval of immunotherapy in the first and second line setting for recurrent/metastatic disease. Various combinations of immunotherapy with targeted therapies, monoclonal antibodies, or human papilloma virus vaccines are also being studied in recurrent/metastatic disease. Currently, programmed death-ligand 1 status is the main marker utilized to assess potential response to immunotherapy. Studies are focused on identifying additional markers, which may help better predict response to immunotherapy for HNSCC patients.

Several imaging modalities are utilized in the diagnosis, treatment, and surveillance of head and neck cancer. First-line imaging remains computed tomography (CT); however, MRI, PET with CT (PET/CT), and ultrasound are often used. In the last decade, several new imaging modalities have been developed that have the potential to improve early detection, modify treatment, decrease treatment morbidity, and augment surveillance. Among these, molecular imaging, lymph node mapping, and adjustments to endoscopic techniques are promising. The present review focuses on existing imaging, novel techniques, and the recent changes to imaging practices within the field.

Margin status in head and neck cancer has important prognostic implications. Currently, resection is based on manual palpation and gross visualization followed by intraoperative specimen or tumor bed–based margin analysis using frozen sections. While generally effective, this protocol has several limitations including margin sampling and close and positive margin re-localization. There is a lack of evidence on the association of use of frozen section analysis with improved survival in head and neck cancer. This article reviews novel technologies in head and neck margin analysis such as 3-dimensional scanning, augmented reality, molecular margins, optical imaging, spectroscopy, and artificial intelligence.

This article examines disparities in head and neck cancer across the cancer care continuum. It provides a public health lens to understand multilevel determinants of health behavior and the importance of social determinants of health. This article reviews the evidence base showing profound differences in incidence, treatment, and survival for patients with head and neck cancer by race, ethnicity, socioeconomic status, and geography. Continued research is needed to understand and address disparities for patients with head and neck cancer.

Head and neck cancer is a potentially traumatizing disease with the potential to impact many of the functions which are core to human life: eating, drinking, breathing, and speaking. Patients with head and neck cancer are disproportionately impacted by socioeconomic challenges, social stigma, and difficult decisions about treatment approaches. Herein, the authors review foundational ethical principles and frameworks to guide care of these patients. The authors discuss specific challenges including shared decision-making and advance care planning. The authors further discuss palliative care with a discussion of the role of surgery as a component of palliation.

Oropharyngeal squamous cell carcinoma (OPSCC) related to human papillomavirus (HPV) infection has better survival outcomes compared to non-HPV-related OPSCC, leading to efforts to de-escalate the intensity of treatment to reduce associated morbidity. This article reviews recent clinical efforts to explore different de-escalation frameworks with a particular emphasis on the emergence of transoral robotic surgery and surgically driven de-escalation approaches. It discusses the current evidence for incorporating surgery into an evolving treatment paradigm for HPV-related OPSCC.

Since its inception, microvascular free tissue transfer has broadened possibilities for oncologic ablation and restoration of form and function. Developments throughout recent decades have resulted in increasing flap success rates and complexity. Advances in technology and knowledge gained from past experiences will continue to improve surgical efficiency, flap success rates, and ultimately, patient outcomes.

Basal cell carcinoma (BCC), cutaneous squamous cell carcinoma (cSCC), and Merkel cell carcinoma (MCC) comprise the majority of nonmelanoma skin cancers. Advances have been made in treatment. Sentinel node biopsy should be considered for locally advanced, clinically node-negative cSCCs and MCCs. BCC patients failing traditional surgery and/or radiation are candidates for systemic hedgehog inhibitor therapy. Immune checkpoint inhibitor treatment is available for patients who failed traditional treatment with surgery and/or radiation or who are not candidates for these modalities. Specifically, cemiplimab is approved for advanced BCC; cemiplimab and pembrolizumab for advanced cSCC; and avelumab, pembrolizumab, and retifanlimab-dlwr for recurrent/metastatic MCC.

The field of endoscopic endonasal surgery is in a constant state of advancement, with an expanding range of applications. Improvement in the diversity of instruments available, along with the increasing proficiency of surgical teams, has enabled the successful endoscopic treatment of complex sinonasal and skull base malignancies. Not only is the overall complication rate reduced by endoscopic approaches, but survival outcomes have also shown promising results when compared to traditional open approaches.

Salivary gland carcinoma is a rare form of head and neck carcinoma, but it comprises a variety of subsites and histologic subtypes that each present with unique clinical courses and management challenges. Preoperative work-up generally consists of fine-needle aspiration cytology and MRI. However, because of the large variety of subtypes, there are often challenges obtaining a histologic diagnosis before surgery. Upfront surgery at the primary site leads to the greatest improvement in survival. Posttreatment surveillance of these patients is important. This article discusses some of the current controversies in the management of salivary gland carcinomas.

Over the last 2 decades, the paradigm of laryngeal cancer management has pivoted toward preserving laryngeal function without sacrificing oncologic outcomes. Transoral laser microsurgery has diminished the role of open laryngeal surgery. For early-stage laryngeal cancer, the common primary modalities are endoscopic laryngeal surgery and narrow field radiation. Total laryngectomy followed by either radiation or chemoradiation is option for advanced laryngeal cancer. In experienced hands and following meticulous patient selection, supracricoid laryngectomy may serve as a viable alternative to total laryngectomy to preserve laryngeal function. Total laryngectomy is still the recommended treatment in those with airway compromise and/or laryngeal dysfunction.

SURGICAL ONCOLOGY CLINICS OF NORTH AMERICA

SERIES OF RELATED INTEREST

Advances in Surgery
https://www.advancessurgery.com
Surgical Clinics of North America
https://www.surgical.theclinics.com
Thoracic Surgery Clinics
https://www.thoracic.theclinics.com

THE CLINICS ARE AVAILABLE ONLINE!
Access your subscription at:
www.theclinics.com

SURGICAL ONCOLOGY
CLINICS OF NORTH AMERICA

Foreword

Evolving Management of Head and Neck Cancers

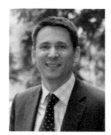

Timothy M. Pawlik, MD, PhD, MPH, MTS, MBA, FACS, FSSO, FRACS (Hon.)
Consulting Editor

This issue of the *Surgical Oncology Clinics of North America* focuses on updates and advancements in the evolving management of head and neck cancers. Cancers arising from the head and neck region comprise broad and often heterogeneous types of malignancies, including melanoma, squamous cell carcinoma, and basal cell cancers— among others. These cancers can drastically impact overall survival, as well as quality of life, as the tumors often arise in areas utilized for breathing, talking, and eating. A relatively common group of cancers, head and neck tumors can be related to viral etiologies (eg, HPV), environmental exposures (eg, tobacco, alcohol, excess sun, and so forth), as well as genetic syndromes (eg, Fanconi anemia and dyskeratosis congenita). Patient prognosis related to head and neck cancers is varied with survival being dictated by stage, as well as histologic subtype. In many instances, treatment of head and neck tumors requires a multidisciplinary approach that involves surgery, medical oncology, and radiation therapy. While advances in robotic and minimally invasive techniques have shifted the surgical approach for many patients with operable disease, recent advances in immunotherapy have revolutionized the treatment of many patients with metastatic disease. In addition, advances in radiation oncology— including the use of proton therapy for certain tumors—have impacted the care of patients with head and neck cancer. As such, the current issue of *Surgical Oncology Clinics of North America* serves to update providers about the latest new clinical approaches to care for patients with head and neck cancer. For this issue, we are lucky to have Dr Sarah L Rohde and Dr Eben L Rosenthal as our guest editors. Dr Rohde is Associate Professor at Vanderbilt School of Medicine, where she is an otolaryngologist specializing in the treatment of patients with medically complex head and neck conditions, many of whom require free-flap surgery. She currently serves as the Associate Division Director of Head and Neck Oncologic Surgery and the Otolaryngology

Surg Oncol Clin N Am 33 (2024) xiii–xiv
https://doi.org/10.1016/j.soc.2024.06.001
1055-3207/24/© 2024 Published by Elsevier Inc.

Surgeon-in-Chief. Her clinical interests include microvascular reconstruction of complex cancer defects and thyroid cancer. Dr Rohde's research focuses on surgical outcomes and efficiency. Dr Eben L Rosenthal is a surgeon-scientist and academic leader who serves as Professor and Chair of the Department of Otolaryngology–Head and Neck Surgery and holds the Barry and Amy Baker Chair in Laryngeal, Head and Neck Research at Vanderbilt. His research interests involve the use of optical imaging techniques to better detect cancer during surgical procedures, and he has initiated multiple clinical trials to improve cancer surgery and assess drug delivery for patients with head and neck cancers.

This issue of *Surgical Oncology Clinics of North America* covers a wide array of topics. In particular, an internationally recognized team of experts reviews various areas, including the role of immunotherapy, novel imaging modalities, state-of-the-art microvascular reconstruction techniques, as well as endoscopic approaches to head and neck cancers. Importantly, the authors also address relevant contemporary issues, such as ethics and palliation, as well as disparities in care for head and neck cancer patients.

I wish to express my sincere gratitude to Drs Rohde and Rosenthal for their work putting together such an amazing group of head and neck cancer experts to contribute to this issue of *Surgical Oncology Clinics of North America*. This team of authors has done a wonderful job highlighting clinically relevant aspects of care for these patients. This issue of *Surgical Oncology Clinics of North America* will help trainees and faculty care for patients with head and neck cancer using the most up-to-date approaches. Thanks again to our guest editors and all the expert authors who contributed to this issue of the *Surgical Oncology Clinics of North America*.

Timothy M. Pawlik, MD, PhD, MPH, MTS, MBA, FACS, FSSO, FRACS (Hon.)
Professor and Chair, Department of Surgery
The Urban Meyer III and
Shelley Meyer Chair for Cancer Research
The Ohio State University
Wexner Medical Center
395 W. 12th Avenue, Suite 670
Columbus, OH 43210, USA

E-mail address:
tim.pawlik@osumc.edu

Preface

Evolving Management of Head and Neck Cancers

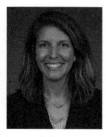 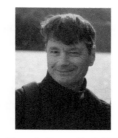

Sarah L. Rohde, MD, MMHC   Eben L. Rosenthal, MD
Editors

Within the broad spectrum of malignancies, head and neck cancer has a unique physical impact because of the social and psychological toll it exacts. In this issue, we embark on a review of new treatment and diagnostic aspects of head and neck cancer—that addresses health disparities, minimally invasive techniques, and new surgical approaches.

The complexities inherent in head and neck cancer demand an interdisciplinary approach, combining surgical intervention with precision (and not so precise) therapuetics and radiation therapy. Decisions made at the time of diagnosis have significant implications for a patient's quality of life, their ability to speak, to eat, to breathe—the very essence of their humanity.

Central to our exploration is the recognition of health disparities that shadow the landscape of cancer care. Disparities in access to health care, in outcomes, and in the burden of disease disproportionately affect certain populations, amplifying the already formidable challenges of a head and neck cancer. We also focus on some minimally invasive techniques for skull base lesions, oropharynx cancers, and laryngeal surgery, as they offer patients the prospect of reduced morbidity, accelerated recovery, and improved functional outcomes. From transoral robotic surgery to endoscopic approaches, we examine the current indications for these techniques and their limitations. We discuss the latest advancements in surgical management, from reconstruction to new techniques for intraoperative surgical imaging.

For Dr Rosenthal and me, our collective vision is shaped by a commitment to excellence, compassion, and collaboration. We are grateful to the authors of the individual articles that bring their wealth of knowledge and experience into a cohesive narrative that informs, inspires, and empowers. Ultimately, we extend our deepest gratitude to the patients and families who entrust us with their care, whose courage and grace

Surg Oncol Clin N Am 33 (2024) xv–xvi
https://doi.org/10.1016/j.soc.2024.05.001
1055-3207/24/© 2024 Published by Elsevier Inc.

surgonc.theclinics.com

illuminate the path forward. We dedicate this issue to them, to our shared journey, and to our collective commitment to improving outcomes.

DISCLOSURES

The authors have no conflicts of interest to disclose.

Sarah L. Rohde, MD, MMHC
Department of Otolaryngology - Head and Neck Surgery
Vanderbilt University Medical Center
Nashville, TN 37232, USA

Eben L. Rosenthal, MD
Department of Otolaryngology–Head and Neck Surgery
Vanderbilt University Medical Center
Nashville, TN 37232, USA

E-mail addresses:
sarah.rohde@vumc.org (S.L. Rohde)
e.rosenthal@vumc.org (E.L. Rosenthal)

Immunotherapy in Head and Neck Cancer
Treatment Paradigms, Future Directions, and Questions

Danielle Fishman, MD[a,b], Jennifer Choe, MD, PhD[b,*]

KEYWORDS

- Immunotherapy • Head and neck cancer • Programmed death-ligand 1-L1
- human papillomavirus

KEY POINTS

- Recent clinical trials have resulted in the approval of immunotherapy for use in both the first- and second-line setting for recurrent or metastatic head and neck squamous cell carcinoma (HNSCC).
- The use of immunotherapy in neoadjuvant setting before surgical resection has shown evidence of pathologic response, with future studies needed to evaluate long-term benefits.
- Areas of future discovery for the use of immunotherapy in HNSCC include combinations with targeted therapies, monoclonal antibodies, and human papillomavirus-specific vaccines in recurrent or metastatic disease.

INTRODUCTION/BACKGROUND/PREVALENCE

Head and neck squamous cell carcinoma (HNSCC) is a diverse group of malignancies from primary origins including oral cavity, oropharynx, and larynx. Overall, HNSCC is the seventh most common malignancy worldwide.[1] In the United States, approximately 51% of cases are locally advanced at time of diagnosis and 15% of cases are metastatic.[1] Common risk factors for HNSCC include tobacco and alcohol use, as well as human papillomavirus (HPV) infection. HPV-related HNSCC more commonly affects the oropharynx. Approximately 30% of oropharyngeal cancers are attributed to HPV, with significant geographic variation and an increased proportion of HPV-positive disease in developed countries.[1] HPV-positive disease is also

[a] Department of Medicine, Vanderbilt University Medical Center, 1161 21st Avenue S, Nashville, TN 37232, USA; [b] Division of Hematology/Oncology, Department of Medicine, Vanderbilt-Ingram Cancer Center, Vanderbilt University Medical Center, 2220 Pierce Avenue, PRB 790, Nashville, TN 37232, USA
* Corresponding author.
E-mail address: jennifer.choe@vumc.org

Surg Oncol Clin N Am 33 (2024) 605–615
https://doi.org/10.1016/j.soc.2024.04.001
1055-3207/24/© 2024 Elsevier Inc. All rights reserved.

surgonc.theclinics.com

associated with increased survival compared with HPV-negative disease.[1] Historically, nasopharyngeal cancer has been considered as a different malignancy in terms of pathology (ie, the role of Ebstein Barr Virus), epidemiology (ie, geographic distribution), and treatment.[2]

In general, survival rates for HNSCC have improved significantly in the setting of advances in surgical resection, radiation therapy, and systemic treatments. The use of immunotherapy (immuno-oncology) for head and neck cancer has changed the treatment landscape, allowing patients who may not be candidates for traditional cytotoxic therapy to have additional treatment options.

USE OF IMMUNOTHERAPY IN FIRST-LINE SETTING FOR RECURRENT OR METASTATIC HEAD AND NECK SQUAMOUS CELL CARCINOMA

The approval of immunotherapy for treatment of recurrent or metastatic HNSCC has resulted in a significant transition in treatment regimens with additional treatment options available to patients who may not tolerate traditional cytotoxic regimens. Before use of immunotherapy, the EXTREME regimen, an intensive regimen including platinum-based therapy with 5-fluorouracil and cetuximab, was standard of care for first-line treatment in recurrent/metastatic HNSCC, but its use was limited by significant associated toxicity.[3] KEYNOTE-048 was a phase 3 study examining outcomes for patients with recurrent ormetastatic HNSCC treated with pembrolizumab monotherapy, pembrolizumab with chemotherapy, and the EXTREME regimen.[4] The study showed improved overall survival (OS) with pembrolizumab alone compared with cetuximab with chemotherapy in patients with programmed death-ligand 1 (PD-L1) combined positive score (CPS) greater than 1.[4] The study also showed improved OS in all patients, regardless of PD-L1 status, treated with pembrolizumab with chemotherapy, compared to cetuximab with chemotherapy.[4] The long-term benefit of I/O based treatment has been confirmed on further analysis with continued survival benefits shown at a 4-year follow-up period.[5] Pembrolizumab monotherapy has also shown improved safety compared to cetuximab with chemotherapy.[4] Based on these results, pembrolizumab with 5-fluorouracil and platinum therapy was approved as first-line treatment for recurrent or metastatic HNSCC, and pembrolizumab monotherapy was approved as first line for patients with PD-L1 positive (CPS >1) disease.

The use of nivolumab and nivolumab plus ipilimumab has also been studied in the first-line setting for recurrent or metastatic HNSCC. CheckMate 714 is a recently published phase 2 trial that did not find a significant benefit in terms of overall response rate (ORR), progression free survival (PFS), or OS for ipilimumab/nivolumab compared with nivolumab used in first-line setting for recurrent or metastatic disease.[6] CheckMate 651 is a study comparing ipilimumab/nivolumab to the EXTREME regimen in the first line setting.[7] The study did not find an OS benefit for patients treated with the immunotherapy regimen, including in a subgroup of patients with CPS greater than 20.[7] However, ipilimumab/nivolumab did show a significantly better safety profile when compared with EXTREME.[7]

Additional immunotherapy agents have also been studied in the first-line setting for recurrent or metastatic HNSCC. The KESTREL trial is a phase 3 study of durvalumab (PD-L1 antibody) and tremelimumab (CTLA-4 antibody) versus the EXTREME regimen in the first-line setting for recurrent or metastatic HNSCC.[8] The study found that the combination of durvalumab and tremelimumab was not superior to EXTREME with regards to OS or median PFS in patients with high PD-L1 expression.[8] The immunotherapy combination did have a significantly lower rate of grade 3or4 adverse events compared with the EXTREME regimen.[8]

USE OF IMMUNOTHERAPY IN PLATINUM-REFRACTORY SETTING FOR LOCALLY RECURRENT OR METASTATIC HEAD AND NECK SQUAMOUS CELL CARCINOMA

Immunotherapy has also been approved for use in the second-line or later setting in treatment of locally recurrent or metastatic HNSCC. The platinum-refractory setting is defined as progression within 6 months of prior curative intent chemoradiation or progression on palliative intent platinum-based treatment.

CheckMate-141 is a phase 3 study evaluating nivolumab versus investigators choice (ie, methotrexate, docetaxel, and cetuximab) in patients with recurrent or metastatic HNSCC previously treated with platinum-based therapy. The study found improved OS and ORR with lower incidence of adverse events in patients treated with nivolumab.[9]

KEYNOTE-012 was a phase 1b study investigating the use of pembrolizumab in patients with recurrent or metastatic HNSCC with evidence of PD-L1 expression (>1% positive by immunohistochemistry).[10] The study found an ORR of 18%, with a modestly higher response rate in patients who were HPV positive (25%) compared with HPV negative (14%).[10] An expansion of this initial study was then performed that included patients regardless of PD-L1 status. The study found a statistically significant improvement in ORR in PD-L1 positive patients (22%) versus PD-L1 negative patients (4%).[11] Pembrolizumab was well-tolerated in this patient population, as 9% of patients experienced grade 3 or higher adverse events.[11] Pembrolizumab was studied further in the phase 2 trial, KEYNOTE-055, in patients previously treated with platinum-based chemotherapy and cetuximab.[12] The study found an ORR of 16% with a median duration of response of 8 months.[12] Response rates were found to be similar in patients regardless of PD-L1 and HPV status. The use of pembrolizumab in the second-line setting was also studied in the phase 3 study, KEYNOTE-040.[13] The study compared the use of pembrolizumab versus investigator's choice (ie, methotrexate, docetaxel, or cetuximab) in the treatment of recurrent/metastatic disease progressed after platinum-based therapy. Pembrolizumab had a modestly improved OS rate and fewer adverse events in this study. Based on the aforementioned study results, both pembrolizumab and nivolumab received Food and Drug Administration approval in 2016 for use in second-line setting for recurrent or metastatic HNSCC.

USE OF IMMUNOTHERAPY IN LOCOREGIONALLY ADVANCED DISEASE
Immunotherapy with Chemotherapy or Radiation

The use of immunotherapy has also been studied in combination with chemoradiation for locally advanced HNSCC. KEYNOTE-412 is phase 3 trial investigating the use of pembrolizumab in combination with concurrent chemotherapy or radiation (CRT) versus placebo in patients with locally advanced HNSCC.[14] The study found a favorable trend towards improved event free survival with the combination of pembrolizumab and concurrent CRT, but this did not achieve statistical significance.[14] The study found favorable trends for all subgroups, except those with CPS score less than 1.[14] The combination of pembrolizumab with CRT did not result in a significant change in adverse events.[14] A phase 3 trial, JAVELIN Head and Neck 100, has also investigated the use of avelumab with CRT in locally advanced HNSCC. The study did not find a prolonged PFS with the addition of avelumb to CRT.[15]

The ideal sequencing of immunotherapy and radiation therapy for locoregionally advanced disease is currently being investigated. By radiating the regional lymph nodes, a critical site for T-cell priming in effective immunotherapy response, it is hypothesized that elective nodal irradiation (ENI) may decrease the overall effectiveness of immunotherapy.[16] A study compared radiation of only the primary tumor versus ENI in mouse models.[16] ENI was found to decrease the systemic immune response of CD4 and CD8 cells with increased metastatic tumor growth.[16] A similar concept could also be applied to surgical lymph node resection, which may also result in blunting of the immunotherapy response. As described in the following, neoadjuvant immunotherapy has been studied before surgical resection. There may be benefit in delayed surgical resection with neoadjuvant immunotherapy to allow time for a systemic immune response. Future studies are needed to evaluate the use of immunotherapy with CRT in locoregionally advanced disease and sequencing of immunotherapy with radiation or surgical resection to optimize treatment outcomes.

Immunotherapy as Neoadjuvant Treatment Before Surgical Resection

Immunotherapy in the neoadjuvant setting has the potential to decrease tumor size before surgical resection, possibly decreasing the extent of surgery required and improving long-term outcomes post-resection. The use of pembrolizumab has been examined in the neoadjuvant setting for resectable HPV-negative HNSCC in a phase 2 study.[17] The study found any level of pathologic response in 44% of patients (16/36 patients) after 2 cycles of pembrolizumab.[17] This notably doubled the pathologic response rate compared with the cohort treated with 1 cycle of the neoadjuvant pembrolizumab. The risk of relapse at 1 year in patients with high-risk disease was also found to be lower than baseline values.[17] KEYNOTE-689 is the largest phase 3 study of neoadjuvant pembrolizumab given for 2 cycles before surgical resection with primary endpoints of major pathologic response and event-free survival.[18] The study has potential to provide important information regarding the use of immunotherapy in the neoadjuvant setting and remains an area of active investigation.

A phase 2 study has also investigated the use of nivolumab and ipilimumab or nivolumab for patients with oral squamous cell carcinoma in the neoadjuvant setting before surgical resection.[19] Pathologic down-staging was found in 53% of patients treated with nivolumab and 69% of patients treated with ipilimumab or nivolumab.[19] A significant proportion of patients had pathologic response (54% with nivolumab and 73% with ipilimumab or nivolumab), however, only a minority had a major pathologic response (7% with nivolumab and 20% with ipilimumab or nivolumab).[19] The use of the combination of ipilimumab and nivolumab in neoadjuvant setting has also been studied in a phase 1 b/2a trial.[20] The study included 32 patients with HNSCC who were treated with 2 doses of immunotherapy (either nivolumab or nivolumab plus a single dose ipilimumab) before surgical resection. A major pathologic response was seen in 35% of patients who received combination therapy using ipilimumab or nivolumab.[20] In general, studies of immunotherapy in the neoadjuvant setting have not showed significant delays or complications with regards to surgical resection. However, the low response rate of current neoadjuvant immunotherapy regimens limits the use of these regimens in standard practice because of risk of progressive disease in the curative intent setting.

The combination of immunotherapy and radiation has also been studied in the neoadjuvant setting before surgical resection. A phase 1b clinical trial of 21 patients with locally advanced HNSCC was conducted evaluating neoadjuvant stereotactic body radiation therapy (SBRT) in combination with nivolumab before definitive surgical resection.[21] The study found the combination of neoadjuvant immunotherapy and radiation resulted in pathologic down-staging in 90% of patients and major pathologic response in 86% of patients.[21] This study found higher rates of down staging and significant pathologic response compared with studies examining neoadjuvant immunotherapy alone. Notably, the study did include mostly patients who were HPV-positive (~76%).[21] The study also included a cohort treated with neoadjuvant SBRT alone, which also resulted in significant and similar major pathologic response of 83% in

HPV-positive patients.[21] Future studies are needed to examine the role of both SBRT and immunotherapy separately versus combined in the neoadjuvant setting before surgical resection.

FUTURE DIRECTIONS
Identifying Responders to Immunotherapy

Future studies are needed to identify which patients with HNSCC respond best to immunotherapy. PD-L1 status, tumor mutational burden (TMB), and HPV status are sub-groups of patients who have been studied with regards to their response to immunotherapy. A meta-analysis including Checkmate 141, KEYNOTE-012, and KEYNOTE-055 found that HPV-positive patients had slightly increased ORR to anti-PD-L1 therapy compared with HPV negative patients (21.9% v. 14.1%).[22] The improved response based on HPV-status was found to be independent of PD-L1 expression and TMB. An increased inflammatory response triggered by HPV-infection may result in increased response to immunotherapy for these patients.

The role of PD-L1 expression has also been studied as an indicator of response in HNSCC to immunotherapy. As described earlier, KEYNOTE-048 found significant survival benefit for patients with recurrent or metastatic HNSCC with PD-L1 CPS greater than 1 treated with pembrolizumab.[4] Additional studies have examined the role of PD-L1 status in long-term survival outcomes. A follow-up study to CheckMate 141 investigated the role of nivolumab in recurrent/metastatic HNSCC treated with prior platinum therapy with analysis performed by PD-L1 status.[23] The study found that OS rates for nivolumab were consistent between PD-L1 expressors and non-expressors at 18-month, 24-month, and 30-month, respectively.[23] Additional studies are needed to evaluate the role of PD-L1 status in both short-term and long-term response to treatment.

TMB has also been studied as a potential marker of response to immunotherapy in patients with HNSCC. A 3-year observational study of 126 patients with HNSCC treated with anti-PD-L1 therapy examined possible markers of increased response.[24] The study found that higher TMB predicted benefit from anti-PD-L1 therapy in HPV-negative cases specifically.[24]

Current studies are focused on identifying possible genetic panels that may predict response to immunotherapy better than PD-L1 status, TMB, or HPV status. A recent study developed a 25-gene panel with results showing improved prediction of response to immunotherapy in HNSCC when compared with TMB alone.[25]

Combination of Immunotherapy and Targeted Therapy

Multiple studies have been completed investigating the combination of immunotherapy and targeted therapies, including epidermal growth factor receptor (EGFR) and vascular endothelial growth factor (VEGF) inhibitors, in the treatment of recurrent or metastatic HNSCC. A phase 2 trial found an ORR of 45% in patients treated with pembrolizumab and cetuximab who had not previously received anti-PD-1 or EGFR therapy.[26] Additionally, the combination of nivolumab and cetuximab has been investigated. The study found an ORR of 22% to this combination despite several of the patients (69%) having previously received anti-PD1 monotherapy or EGFR therapy.[27]

The use of VEGF inhibitors and immunotherapy has also been studied, with the thought that inhibition of angiogenesis could add to response of immunotherapy. A phase 1 b or 2 study of lenvatinib and pembrolizumab was completed in various solid malignancies, including renal cell, urothelial cancer, endometrial cancer, melanoma, non-small cell lung cancer, and HNSCC.[28] The study included 22 patients with

HNSCC with an ORR of 36% and a reasonable safety profile.[28] Based on these results, a phase 3 study investigated the use of pembrolizumab and lenvatinib versus pembrolizumab monotherapy in the first-line setting for recurrent or metastatic HNSCC with CPS greater than 1.[29] Interim analysis results were recently released, and the combination did not result in OS benefit for patients.[30]

A phase 2 study published in 2023 also investigated the use of pembrolizumab and cabozantinib, a multiple tyrosine kinase inhibitor targeting mesenchymal-epithelial transition pathway and vascular endothelial growth factor receptor 2, in recurrent ormetastatic HNSCC with no prior treatment with immunotherapy.[31] The study included 31 patients and found an ORR of 45.2% and 1-year PFS of 51.8%. It is notable that 41% of patients in this study required dose-reduction in cabozantinib because of toxicity.[31]

New targeted therapies are also being studied in combination with immunotherapy in HNSCC. Evorpacept (ALX148) works by binding to CD47, which is an immune-suppressing cell surface protein that acts as a "don't eat me" signal and has increased expression in many solid and hematologic malignancies.[32] By blocking this signaling pathway, the immune response is increased by macrophages, dendritic cells, and CD8 T-cells. A phase 1 study (ASPEN-01) included patients with HNSCC who received evorpacept in combination with pembrolizumab.[32] The study found an overall response of 20% (4 patients) in the 20 patients with HNSCC treated with evorpacept and pembrolizumab.[32] The study also found a favorable safety profile for the new agent.

Combination of Monoclonal Antibodies and Immunotherapy

Monoclonal antibodies are an additional treatment modality being studied in combination with immunotherapy in treatment of HNSCC. Monalizumab is a monoclonal antibody targeting the natural killer group 2 receptor on Natural Killer (NK) cells that is currently being studied in recurrent or metastatic HNSCC.[33] A phase 2 study, the UPSTREAM study, showed initial limited response to monalizumab therapy with median progression of 1.7 months.[33] However, the use of monalizumab in combination with immunotherapy (ie, durvalumab) is currently in process. An additional monoclonal antibody currently being studied in HNSCC is feladilumab, an inducible T-cell costimulatory agonist antibody, in combination with pembrolizumab in the first-line treatment of PD-L1 positive recurrent or metastatic disease.[34] Monoclonal antibodies against LAG-3 have also been studied in combination with nivolumab in a variety of solid malignancies, including a sub-group of patients with HNSCC.[35] LAG-3 is a cell surface receptor that is thought to play an important role in immune system regulation, similarly to PD-L1 and CTLA-4, by inhibiting the common pathway of CD4 and CD8 activation.[36] In contrast, soluble LAG-3 (sLAG3) is a cleaved form of LAG-3 to be shed from the cell membrane to activate immune stimulatory functions by activating antigen presenting cells and subsequent CD8 + effector T-cell function. Soluble LAG-3 protein eftilagimod alpha with pembrolizumab has demonstrated promising results in the TACTI-002 phase 2 trial in recurrent or metastatic HNSCC with 27.0% ORR in the intent-to-treat population.[37] Monoclonal antibodies targeting CD155/TIGIT in combination with PD-L1 inhibition have been studied in mouse models.[38] TIGIT (T-cell immunoglobulin and ITIM domain) is an additional immunosuppressing molecule expressed on activated T-cell subtypes and NK cells that binds CD155 and is thought to possibly act synergistically with PD-L1 signaling. A study in mouse models showed that combined blockage of CD155/TIGIT and PD/PD-L1 resulted in significantly decreased tumor growth.[38]

Additionally, new bifunctional antibodies are being developed and studied in combination with immunotherapy. BCA101 is a bifunctional fusion antibody that targets both EGFR and TGFβ simultaneously.[39] It has been studied in mouse models of HNSCC with immunotherapy and showed durable response.[39] There is an ongoing phase 1 study investigating BCA101 and pembrolizumab as first-line treatment for recurrent or metastatic HNSCC with PD-L1 CPS score greater than 1.[39] Interim analysis from the study has shown a manageable safety profile for the combination. The ORR was found to be 48%, with higher response rates in HPV-negative patients (65% for HPV negative vs 18% for HPV positive), and median PFS was 4.8 months.[40] Petosemtamab is an additional bifunctional antibody being studied in HNSCC.[41] This agent targets both EGFR and LGR5 (leucine-rich, repeat-containing, G-protein coupled receptor 5), a receptor expressed on cancer stem cells.[41] It was found to have an ORR of approximately 36% and MPS of 5.0 months in a cohort of HNSCC patients with the majority receiving prior treatment with checkpoint inhibitors and platinum-based therapy.[41] Further studies are needed for these monoclonal antibody agents as monotherapy and in combination with standard treatment in larger randomized trials.

Combination of Human Papillomavirus Targeting Vaccine and Immunotherapy

For HPV-positive HNSCC, the combination of HPV vaccines and immunotherapy is also being studied. ISA101 is an HPV-16 peptide vaccine that has been utilized in combination with nivolumab for patients with recurrent HPV-16 positive cancer.[42] The study found an ORR of 33% with median duration of response of 11.2 months.[42] A randomized trial is ongoing comparing nivolumab with ISA101 versus nivolumab monotherapy. The use of HPV targeting vaccines is also being studied in combination with pembrolizumab. A phase 2 study is underway evaluating BNT113, an HPV vaccine, in combination with pembrolizumab versus pembrolizumab monotherapy in first-line treatment of recurrent or metastatic HPV-16 and PD-1 positive (CPS >1) HNSCC.[43]

Future Role for Chimeric Antigen Receptor-T in Treatment of Head and Neck Squamous Cell Carcinoma

A developing treatment modality being studied for HNSCC is the use of Chimeric Antigen Receptor-T (CAR-T) cell therapy, in which immune cells are generated to target specific markers on the surface of tumor cells. In vitro studies have shown that human epidermal growth factor receptor 2 could be a potential target for CAR-T therapy in HNSCC.[44] CD70 is an additional target that has been specifically identified for possible use in CAR-T in HNSCC.[45] Recently, results were published for a T-cell therapy targeting melanoma-associated antigen 4.[46] The study found a 50% response rate in a cohort of patients with HNSCC, ovarian, and urothelial cancer with an acceptable safety profile.[46] The agent is also currently being studied in combination with nivolumab in HNSCC patients.

SUMMARY

Immunotherapy in the treatment of HNSCC remains a growing and evolving field. Recent studies have resulted in the approval of immunotherapy, in combination with chemotherapy or as monotherapy, in the first-and second-line setting for recurrent or metastatic disease. The use of immunotherapy in the neoadjuvant setting has the potential to decrease the extent of surgical resection required. Studies have shown pathologic response in this setting, however, future studies are needed to improve response rates to offset the risk of progression in the curative setting and evaluate long-term outcomes. The use of immunotherapy with various treatment modalities (targeted therapies, monoclonal antibodies, and HPV vaccines), as well as better identifying patients, who may benefit from immunotherapy continue to be an area of future discovery.

CLINICS CARE POINTS

- Pembrolizumab with 5-fluorouracil and platinum therapy is approved as first-line treatment for recurrent or metastatic HNSCC with any CPS score, and pembrolizumab monotherapy is approved as first line treatment for patients with PD-L1 positive (CPS >1) disease. No other immune checkpoint inhibitors are approved in first-line therapy for HNSCC.

- Both pembrolizumab and nivolumab have received Food and Drug Administration approval for use in the second-line (platinum-refractory) setting for recurrent or metastatic HNSCC. There are no other FDA-approved immune checkpoint inhibitors for platinum-refractory HNSCC.

- Currently, PD-L1 status is the main marker utilized to predict individual response to immunotherapy in HNSCC with ongoing studies evaluating additional potential predictors of response (i.e., tumor mutation burden, HPV status)

DISCLOSURE

D. Fishman has no disclosures. J. Choe has served on a scientific expert panel for Merck Sharpe & Dohme and as an advisory board member for Coherus Biosciences, Exelixis, Eisai, Regeneron-Sanofi, and receives institutional research funding from Genmab A/S, Merck Sharpe & Dohme, ALX Oncology, Coherus Biosciences, Rakuten, and Genentech/Roche.

REFERENCES

1. Barsouk A, Aluru JS, Rawla P, et al. Epidemiology, Risk Factors, and Prevention of Head and Neck Squamous Cell Carcinoma. Med Sci 2023;11(2):42.
2. Cantù G. Nasopharyngeal carcinoma. A "different" head and neck tumour. Part A: from histology to staging. Acta Otorhinolaryngol Ital 2023;43(2):85–98.
3. Vermorken JB, Mesia R, Rivera F, et al. Platinum-based chemotherapy plus cetuximab in head and neck cancer. N Engl J Med 2008;359(11):1116–27.
4. Burtness B, Harrington KJ, Greil R, et al. Pembrolizumab alone or with chemotherapy versus cetuximab with chemotherapy for recurrent or metastatic squamous cell carcinoma of the head and neck (KEYNOTE-048): a randomised, open-label, phase 3 study. Lancet 2019;394(10212):1915–28.
5. Harrington KJ, Burtness B, Greil R, et al. Pembrolizumab With or Without Chemotherapy in Recurrent or Metastatic Head and Neck Squamous Cell Carcinoma: Updated Results of the Phase III KEYNOTE-048 Study. J Clin Oncol 2023; 41(4):790–802.
6. Harrington KJ, Ferris RL, Gillison M, et al. Efficacy and Safety of Nivolumab Plus Ipilimumab vs Nivolumab Alone for Treatment of Recurrent or Metastatic Squamous Cell Carcinoma of the Head and Neck: The Phase 2 CheckMate 714 Randomized Clinical Trial. JAMA Oncol 2023;9(6):779–89.
7. Haddad RI, Harrington K, Tahara M, et al. Nivolumab Plus Ipilimumab Versus EXTREME Regimen as First-Line Treatment for Recurrent/Metastatic Squamous Cell Carcinoma of the Head and Neck: The Final Results of CheckMate 651. J Clin Oncol 2023;41(12):2166–80.

8. Psyrri A, Fayette J, Harrington K, et al. Durvalumab with or without tremelimumab versus the EXTREME regimen as first-line treatment for recurrent or metastatic squamous cell carcinoma of the head and neck: KESTREL, a randomized, open-label, phase III study. Ann Oncol 2023;34(3):262–74.

9. Gillison ML, Blumenschein G Jr, Fayette J, et al. CheckMate 141: 1-Year Update and Subgroup Analysis of Nivolumab as First-Line Therapy in Patients with Recurrent/Metastatic Head and Neck Cancer. Oncol 2018;23(9):1079–82.

10. Seiwert TY, Burtness B, Mehra R, et al. Safety and clinical activity of pembrolizumab for treatment of recurrent or metastatic squamous cell carcinoma of the head and neck (KEYNOTE-012): an open-label, multicentre, phase 1b trial. Lancet Oncol 2016;17(7):956–65.

11. Chow LQM, Haddad R, Gupta S, et al. Antitumor Activity of Pembrolizumab in Biomarker-Unselected Patients With Recurrent and/or Metastatic Head and Neck Squamous Cell Carcinoma: Results From the Phase Ib KEYNOTE-012 Expansion Cohort. J Clin Oncol 2016;34(32):3838–45.

12. Bauml J, Seiwert TY, Pfister DG, et al. Pembrolizumab for Platinum- and Cetuximab-Refractory Head and Neck Cancer: Results From a Single-Arm, Phase II Study. J Clin Oncol 2017;35(14):1542–9.

13. Cohen EEW, Soulières D, Le Tourneau C, et al. Pembrolizumab versus methotrexate, docetaxel, or cetuximab for recurrent or metastatic head-and-neck squamous cell carcinoma (KEYNOTE-040): a randomised, open-label, phase 3 study. Lancet 2019;393(10167):156–67 [published correction appears in Lancet. 2019 Jan 12;393(10167):132].

14. Machiels JP, Tao Y, Burtness B, et al. Pembrolizumab given concomitantly with chemoradiation and as maintenance therapy for locally advanced head and neck squamous cell carcinoma: KEYNOTE-412. Future Oncol 2020;16(18): 1235–43.

15. Lee NY, Ferris RL, Psyrri A, et al. Avelumab plus standard-of-care chemoradiotherapy versus chemoradiotherapy alone in patients with locally advanced squamous cell carcinoma of the head and neck: a randomised, double-blind, placebo-controlled, multicentre, phase 3 trial. Lancet Oncol 2021;22(4):450–62.

16. Darragh LB, Gadwa J, Pham TT, et al. Elective nodal irradiation mitigates local and systemic immunity generated by combination radiation and immunotherapy in head and neck tumors. Nat Commun 2022;13(1):7015.

17. Uppaluri R, Campbell KM, Egloff AM, et al. Neoadjuvant and Adjuvant Pembrolizumab in Resectable Locally Advanced, Human Papillomavirus-Unrelated Head and Neck Cancer: A Multicenter, Phase II Trial. Clin Cancer Res 2020; 26(19):5140–52 [published correction appears in Clin Cancer Res. 2021 Jan 1;27(1):357].

18. Uppaluri R, Lee N, Westra W, et al. KEYNOTE-689: Phase 3 study of adjuvant and neoadjuvant pembrolizumab combined with standard of care (SOC) in patients with resectable, locally advanced head and neck squamous cell carcinoma. J Clin Oncol 2019;37. https://doi.org/10.1200/JCO.2019.37.15_suppl.TPS6090.

19. Schoenfeld JD, Hanna GJ, Jo VY, et al. Neoadjuvant Nivolumab or Nivolumab Plus Ipilimumab in Untreated Oral Cavity Squamous Cell Carcinoma: A Phase 2 Open-Label Randomized Clinical Trial. JAMA Oncol 2020;6(10):1563–70.

20. Vos JL, Elbers JBW, Krijgsman O, et al. Neoadjuvant immunotherapy with nivolumab and ipilimumab induces major pathological responses in patients with head and neck squamous cell carcinoma. Nat Commun 2021;12(1):7348.

21. Leidner R, Crittenden M, Young K, et al. Neoadjuvant immunoradiotherapy results in high rate of complete pathological response and clinical to pathological

downstaging in locally advanced head and neck squamous cell carcinoma. J Immunother Cancer 2021;9(5):e002485.

22. Wang J, Sun H, Zeng Q, et al. HPV-positive status associated with inflamed immune microenvironment and improved response to anti-PD-1 therapy in head and neck squamous cell carcinoma. Sci Rep 2019;9(1):13404.

23. Ferris RL, Blumenschein G Jr, Fayette J, et al. Nivolumab vs investigator's choice in recurrent or metastatic squamous cell carcinoma of the head and neck: 2-year long-term survival update of CheckMate 141 with analyses by tumor PD-L1 expression. Oral Oncol 2018;81:45–51.

24. Hanna GJ, Lizotte P, Cavanaugh M, et al. Frameshift events predict anti-PD-1/L1 response in head and neck cancer. JCI Insight 2018;3(4):e98811.

25. Huang Y, Liao J, Liang F, et al. A 25-gene panel predicting the benefits of immunotherapy in head and neck squamous cell carcinoma. Int Immunopharmacol 2022;110:108846.

26. Sacco AG, Chen R, Worden FP, et al. Pembrolizumab plus cetuximab in patients with recurrent or metastatic head and neck squamous cell carcinoma: an open-label, multi-arm, non-randomised, multicentre, phase 2 trial. Lancet Oncol 2021; 22(6):883–92.

27. Chung CH, Bonomi M, Steuer CE, et al. Concurrent Cetuximab and Nivolumab as a Second-Line or beyond Treatment of Patients with Recurrent and/or Metastatic Head and Neck Squamous Cell Carcinoma: Results of Phase I/II Study. Cancers 2021;13(5):1180.

28. Taylor MH, Lee CH, Makker V, et al. Phase IB/II Trial of Lenvatinib Plus Pembrolizumab in Patients With Advanced Renal Cell Carcinoma, Endometrial Cancer, and Other Selected Advanced Solid Tumors. J Clin Oncol 2020;38(11):1154–63 [published correction appears in J Clin Oncol. 2020 Aug 10;38(23):2702].

29. Siu LL, Burtness B, Cohen E, et al. Phase III LEAP-010 study: first-line pembrolizumab with or without lenvatinib in recurrent/metastatic (R/M) head and neck squamous cell carcinoma (HNSCC). J Clin Oncol 2020;38. https://doi.org/10.1200/JCO.2020.38.15_suppl.TPS6589.

30. Merck and Eisai provide update on phase 3 LEAP-010 trial evaluating Keytruda® (PEMBROLIZUMAB) plus LENVIMA® (lenvatinib) in patients with certain types of recurrent or metastatic head and neck squamous cell carcinoma. Merck.com. 2023. Available at: https://www.merck.com/news/merck-and-eisai-provide-update-on-phase-3-leap-010-trial-evaluating-keytruda-pembrolizumab-plus-lenvima-lenvatinib-in-patients-with-certain-types-of-recurrent-or-metastatic-head-and-ne/. [Accessed 14 January 2024].

31. Saba NF, Steuer CE, Ekpenyong A, et al. Pembrolizumab and cabozantinib in recurrent metastatic head and neck squamous cell carcinoma: a phase 2 trial. Nat Med 2023;29(4):880–7.

32. Lakhani NJ, Chow LQM, Gainor JF, et al. Evorpacept alone and in combination with pembrolizumab or trastuzumab in patients with advanced solid tumours (ASPEN-01): a first-in-human, open-label, multicentre, phase 1 dose-escalation and dose-expansion study. Lancet Oncol 2021;22(12):1740–51.

33. Galot R, Le Tourneau C, Saada-Bouzid E, et al. A phase II study of monalizumab in patients with recurrent/metastatic squamous cell carcinoma of the head and neck: The I1 cohort of the EORTC-HNCG-1559 UPSTREAM trial. Eur J Cancer 2021. https://doi.org/10.1016/j.ejca.2021.09.003.

34. Hansen AR, Stanton T, Hong M, et al. INDUCE-3: A randomized, double-blind study of GSK3359609 (GSK609), an inducible T-cell co-stimulatory (ICOS) agonist antibody, plus pembrolizumab (PE) versus placebo (PL) plus PE for

first-line treatment of PD-L1-positive recurrent/metastatic head and neck squamous cell carcinoma (R/M HNSCC). J Clin Oncol 2020;38:TPS6591. https://doi.org/10.1200/JCO.2020.38.15_suppl.TPS6591.

35. An Investigational Immuno-therapy Study to Assess the Safety, Tolerability and Effectiveness of Anti-LAG-3 With and Without Anti-PD-1 in the Treatment of Solid Tumors. Clinicaltrials.gov. 2023. Available at: https://www.clinicaltrials.gov/study/NCT01968109#publications. [Accessed 9 January 2024].

36. Chocarro L, Blanco E, Zuazo M, et al. Understanding LAG-3 Signaling. Int J Mol Sci 2021;22(10):5282.

37. Doger de Spéville B, Felip E, Forster M, et al. Final results from TACTI-002 Part C: A phase II study of eftilagimod alpha (soluble LAG-3 protein) and pembrolizumab in patients with metastatic 2nd line head and neck squamous cell carcinoma unselected for PD-L1. J Clin Oncol 2023;41:6029. https://doi.org/10.1200/JCO.2023.41.16_suppl.6029.

38. Mao L, Xiao Y, Yang QC, et al. TIGIT/CD155 blockade enhances anti-PD-L1 therapy in head and neck squamous cell carcinoma by targeting myeloid-derived suppressor cells. Oral Oncol 2021;121:105472.

39. Boreddy SR, Nair R, Pandey PK, et al. BCA101 Is a Tumor-Targeted Bifunctional Fusion Antibody That Simultaneously Inhibits EGFR and TGFβ Signaling to Durably Suppress Tumor Growth. Cancer Res 2023;83(11):1883–904.

40. Hanna G.J., Kaczmar J.M., Zandberg D.P., et al., Dose expansion results of the bifunctional EGFR/TGFβ inhibitor BCA101 with pembrolizumab in patients with recurrent, metastatic head and neck squamous cell carcinoma. 2023 ASCO Annual Meeting. Abstract 6005. Chicago, IL. Presented June 5, 2023.

41. Cohen EE, Fayette J, Daste A, et al. Abstract CT012: Clinical activity of MCLA-158 (petosemtamab), an IGG1 bispecific antibody targeting EGFR and LGR5, in advanced head and neck squamous cell cancer (HNSCC). American Association for Cancer Research. 2023. Available at: https://aacrjournals.org/cancerres/article/83/8_Supplement/CT012/725328/Abstract-CT012-Clinical-activity-of-MCLA-158. [Accessed 14 January 2024].

42. Sousa LG, Rajapakshe K, Rodriguez Canales J, et al. ISA101 and nivolumab for HPV-16+ cancer: updated clinical efficacy and immune correlates of response. J Immunother Cancer 2022;10(2):e004232.

43. A clinical trial investigating the safety, tolerability, and therapeutic effects of BNT113 in combination with pembrolizumab versus pembrolizumab alone for patients with a form of head and neck cancer positive for human papilloma virus 16 and expressing the protein PD-L1 - Full Text View. ClinicalTrials.gov. 2020. Available at: https://classic.clinicaltrials.gov/ct2/show/NCT04534205. [Accessed 9 January 2024].

44. Warren E., Liu H.-C., Porter C.E., et al., Overexpression of HER2 in head and neck cancer represents a potential target for T cell immunotherapy abstract. In: Proceedings of the American Association for Cancer Research Annual Meeting 2019. 2019 Mar 29-Apr 3; Atlanta, GA.

45. Park YP, Jin L, Bennett KB, et al. CD70 as a target for chimeric antigen receptor T cells in head and neck squamous cell carcinoma. Oral Oncol 2018;78:145–50.

46. Next-generation TCR T-cell therapy (ADP-A2M4CD8) demonstrates strong efficacy in a broad range of solid tumors; Adaptimmune presents data update from its surpass trial at Esmo. Adaptimmune. 2023. Available at: https://www.adaptimmune.com/investors-and-media/news-center/press-releases/detail/251/next-generation-tcr-t-cell-therapy-adp-a2m4cd8. [Accessed 14 January 2024].

Imaging Modalities for Head and Neck Cancer
Present and Future

Gabriel A. Hernandez-Herrera, BS[a], Gabriela A. Calcano, BS[a],
Alex A. Nagelschneider, MD[b], David M. Routman, MD[c],
Kathryn M. Van Abel, MD[a,*]

KEYWORDS

- Imaging • Head and neck cancer • Squamous cell carcinoma • CT • MRI
- FDG-PET/CT • US • Novel techniques

KEY POINTS

- Computed tomography (CT), MRI, PET/CT, and ultrasound remain the foundational imaging techniques for head and neck cancer (HNC).
- Several new imaging modalities have the potential to augment and, in some cases, replace traditional techniques.
- Reviewing the recent changes to imaging practices within the field is critical for improving localization of clinically undetectable HNC.

INTRODUCTION

Head and Neck cancer (HNC) predominantly arises from mucosal or cutaneous epithelium, with squamous cell carcinoma (SCC) accounting for over 90% of all HNC.[1] The remainder of HNC includes a wide variety of subsites and histologies, including but not limited to, thyroid, salivary, other skin malignancies, and more rare diseases. Therefore, the head and neck (H&N) oncologist must be well informed about the imaging technologies available for both evaluation and surveillance. Most patients with HNC undergo at least 1 imaging study during evaluation for evaluation of primary, regional, or distant disease. Common techniques used for HNC imaging include computed tomography (CT), magnetic resonance imaging (MRI), positron emission tomography (PET)/CT, and ultrasound (US). Imaging plays a crucial role in diagnosis,

Financial material & support: Internal departmental funding was utilized without commercial sponsorship or support.
^a Department of Otolaryngology–Head and Neck Surgery, Mayo Clinic; ^b Department of Radiology, Mayo Clinic; ^c Department of Radiation Oncology, Mayo Clinic
* Corresponding author. 200 1st Street SW, Rochester, MN
E-mail address: vanabel.kathryn@mayo.edu

staging, assessing response to treatment, and surveillance. Imaging studies help elucidate the extent of a primary tumor, the burden of regional lymphadenopathy, and the presence or absence of distant disease to inform staging and serve as the foundation for treatment decision making. Although imaging modality selection for HNC is complex and multifactorial, cost and availability may drive selection at various stages of disease.

Although conventional imaging with CT or PET/CT has been the standard of care for disease surveillance, recent studies have shown that blood tests might be more sensitive and specific for early detection. Liquid biopsies offer a non-invasive route for tumor detection and have demonstrated great potential in monitoring disease, especially for human papillomavirus (HPV)-associated oropharyngeal squamous cell carcinoma [HPV(+)OPSCC].[2] In addition, multicancer early detection (MCED) tests, which are now commercially available, offer the ability to test the blood of healthy asymptomatic individuals for a myriad of cancers.[3-5] Although false positives for HPV cancers (a positive biomarker result with a negative clinical and/or imaging examination) occur in less than 2% of patients, it is still unclear how to address this issue.[6,7] This underscores the need to add new imaging modalities to complement our ability to localize and eradicate early cancers, minimal residual disease, and recurrences.

In this review, the authors discuss briefly standard imaging modalities for HNC and examine the current evidence for novel imaging methods considering emerging literature on early diagnostic strategies. Ultimately, we seek to inform future directions on a comprehensive diagnostic toolkit.

CURRENT IMAGING TECHNIQUES
Computed Tomography

CT is often the first-line imaging modality for assessing and diagnosing HNC in adults. Due to its widespread availability, rapid results, and relatively low cost, CT scans serve to quickly locate and characterize new masses, especially when used in conjunction with PET.[8-10] CT uses an X-ray source and detectors to create cross-sectional images based on the different attenuation characteristics of different tissues.[11] Due to its capability for high spatial resolution, CT allows for detection of subtle findings such as early osseous erosion.[12] Evaluation of the latter may be facilitated by the puffed-cheek technique and in the setting of metal orthodontic implants, noise reduction through the open mouth technique is especially beneficial for tumors on the mobile tongue, retromolar trigone, and palatine tonsil (**Fig. 1**).[13,14]

CT can be used to further investigate soft tissue pathology when combined with intravenous (IV) iodinated contrast. The use of IV contrast in CT allows for more accurate assessment of tumor details that impact staging and prognosis such as size, involvement of adjacent structures, and assessment of adjacent vascularity, which is critical for surgical planning. Generally, CT has a reported sensitivity and specificity of 68% and 69% in the detection of primary HNC, and 63% and 80% for recurrent tumors, respectively.[15] Its importance in surgical planning is more difficult to quantify, but it is critical for planning the surgical procedure and the reconstruction (vessel availability).

Notably, utilizing CT scanning in pre-operative evaluations of nodal metastasis is superior to physical examination findings alone.[16,17] The use of contrast increases CT sensitivity for nodal tissue substantially, providing further insight into regional metastasis.[18] Still, PET/CT was found to be more specific and more accurate, with a higher negative predictive value in patients with OPSCC.[18] In order to clinically stage HNC, it is critical to investigate metastatic lymph nodes and consider the number, laterality,

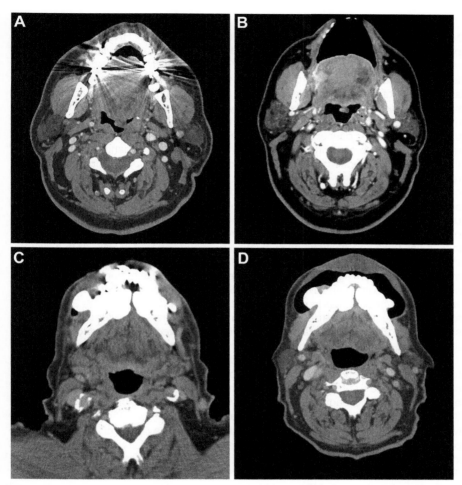

Fig. 1. Computed tomography (CT) images demonstrating open mouth and puffed-cheek techniques. (*A*) Case of a 64-year-old male with a right oral tongue squamous cell carcinoma (SCC) obscured by amalgam artifacts. (*B*) Improved visualization of the tumor with the open mouth technique. (*C, D*) Case of a 79-year-old male presenting with a right mandibular alveolar SCC on the anterior and superior surface of a right labial mandibular exostosis. A soft tissue prominence is visualized on images obtained with the puffed-cheek technique.

size, architecture (cystic vs solid), and presence or absence of extranodal extension.[19] In a systematic review and meta-analysis, Sun and colleagues found the use of CT for cervical lymph node metastasis to be 77% sensitive and 85% specific, comparable to findings on MRI which were 72% and 84%, respectively.[20]

The National Comprehensive Cancer Network (NCCN) Clinical Practice Guidelines in Oncology for Head and Neck Cancers Version 2.2024 recommend the use of CT for initial imaging of the primary tumor site and evaluation of lymph node metastasis.[21] Primary HNCs frequently metastasize to the lungs, liver, and bones and while CT is suitable for evaluation of distant metastatic disease, 18F-fluoro-2-deoxyglucose (FDG)-PET/CT is generally preferred.[21,22]

Magnetic Resonance Imaging

MRI with and without contrast is also used for initial imaging of HNC primary sites.[23] In comparison to CT, MRI confers superior soft tissue resolution allowing for more accurate delineation of extent of tumor invasion.[24] Additionally, MRI is known to be superior to CT in evaluation of the marrow space as well as nerves, allowing for more accurate assessment of bone marrow involvement, perineural tumor spread, and intracranial spread of disease.[25,26] The presence of any of the aforementioned may impact treatment course dramatically, as is the case for mandibular bone marrow invasion where it upstages oral cavity cancers to tumor stage (T) 4 disease.[27] Similarly, nasopharyngeal malignancies are preferably assessed with MRI as it offers enhanced assessment of the skull base for bone marrow invasion and intracranial spread.[28] The most common reason for MRI imaging (rather than CT) is assessment of perineural invasion, especially in the context of cranial nerve symptoms, suspected bone marrow invasion, sinonasal malignancies, and in tumors abutting the skull base. MRI has a sensitivity of 97% and specificity of 61% in detecting bone marrow invasion of the mandible or maxilla in patients with squamous cell carcinoma of the oral cavity (OCSCC).[29] Similarly, it has 95% sensitivity when evaluating perineural spread in HNC.[30] In a systematic review and meta-analysis, Cho and colleagues found MRI to be 88% sensitive for the detection of cartilage invasion in patients with laryngeal or hypopharyngeal cancer, a significantly higher sensitivity than CT (66%).[31] However, no significant differences were found when comparing specificities between the 2, 81% versus 90% for MRI and CT, respectively. In the setting of primary nasopharyngeal tumors, MRI has a sensitivity of 100%, a significant increase when compared to endoscopic examination alone (88%), while its 92% specificity seems to be limited by lymphoid hyperplasia.[32]

Evaluation of H&N metastatic lymph nodes with MRI has improved largely due to technological innovation, where fat-suppression sequences and gadolinium enhancement have made it, at the very least, noninferior to CT in evaluation of regional disease.[33] Liao and colleagues reported an MRI sensitivity of 65% and a specificity of 81% for the detection of lymph node metastasis in patients with HNC and clinically lymph node stage (cN) 0 necks.[34] The eighth edition of the American Joint Committee on Cancer (AJCC) added extranodal extension criteria for N stages, underscoring its importance in risk stratifying patients with head and neck squamous cell carcinomas (HNSCC), especially for HPV(−)OPSCC.[35] In a systematic review and meta-analysis by Park and colleagues MRI pooled sensitivities and specificities were 60% and 96%, respectively, in detecting extranodal extension in patients with HNSCC.[36] However, evaluation of patients with confirmed nodal metastases from carcinoma of unknown primary sites (CUP) remains difficult, especially for palatine tonsil primaries (Fig. 2).[37–39] Lee and colleagues recently described an MRI radiomics-based approach that significantly improves the sensitivity of detecting occult palatine tonsil SCC primaries, reporting 90% sensitivity from the apparent diffusion coefficient model alone and an improvement of 34.6% over that of conventional MRI.[40]

Although advantages of using MRI for HNC are well documented, there are drawbacks. MRI is a more limited resource in most centers compared to CT. Additionally, MRI requires patients to hold still for extended periods of time, up to several minutes for certain sequences, with even minimal patient motion can result in artifacts that may impact the radiologist's ability to adequately assess both the primary tumor and metastatic nodes.[41] Additionally, overall extent of disease is likely to be overestimated on MRI because of associated peritumoral edema and inflammatory changes, especially on T2-weighted images.[42,43] Higher costs associated with MRI scanners along with limited availability in certain regions may limit its use[44,45] In addition, geopolitical

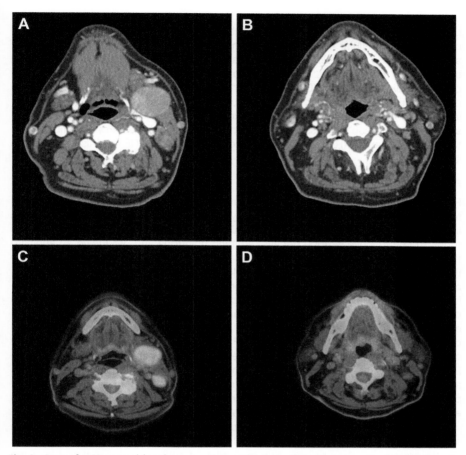

Fig. 2. Case of a 62-year-old male presenting with cervicallymphadenopathy in his left neck. Endoscopy did not reveal any oropharyngeal mass. CT evaluation (*A, B*) showed multiple abnormal and pathologically enlarged lymph nodes in levels II through IV on their left cervical chain, suggesting metastatic disease from a carcinoma of unknown primary sites. Ultrasound (US)-guided core biopsy revealed metastatic p16-positive SCC. Subsequent PET/CT (*C, D*) imaging showed multiple 18-F-fluoro-2-deoxyglucose-avid lymph nodes but failed to identify a site of primary disease.

circumstances have tightened an already limited semiconductor supply, potentially contributing to continuously elevated health care costs, which would impact MRI technology more than others.[46,47] Zero boil-off machines, equipped with refrigeration systems that allow the recondensation of helium and significantly decrease refill frequency, may result in decreased maintenance costs associated with MRI machines by cutting on helium refill expenses.[48]

The application of harmonic or wave-like mechanical forces during MRI provides a non-invasive method to measure tissue stiffness.[49] This technique, known as magnetic resonance elastography (MRE), serves to quantify the mechanical properties of tissues by mapping shear waves displacement patterns using phase-contrast MRI, thereby providing valuable insights into pathologic states including tumor detection and disease characterization.[50] In a review of the biomechanics and biophysics of cancer cells, Suresh highlights increased tissue stiffness driven by a change in extracellular matrix composition and cell-cell adhesion dynamics.[51] MRE shows promising applications in the H&N, as showcased by a recent study evaluating the elasticity of metastatic cervical lymph nodes in patients with HNSCC using diffusion-weighed imaging (DWI)-based virtual MRE. Jung and colleagues found the mean, median, and maximum elasticity values of metastatic lymph nodes to be significantly higher than those of benign lymph nodes on virtual MRE.[52] Similarly, deep and subcutaneous tissue stiffness quantification serves as an indicator of neck fibrosis after radiation therapy (RT).[53] However, studies evaluating MRE for this purpose are lacking.

Positron Emission Tomography

PET scans are nuclear imaging tests that make use of a radioactive isotope attached to a biologically active molecule, commonly FDG, creating a radiotracer that provides insight into a metabolic process.[54] Usually administrated through an intravenous route, the radioactive isotope decays, emitting positrons and producing an annihilation event along with 2 gamma rays that travel in opposite directions detected by the scanner.[55,56] Gamma ray detection allows the scanner to compute their origin, creating a 3-dimensional image of tracer concentration within the body along metabolically active tissues.[56] Importantly, this technology is ideally used with CT scans to register the PET scan to the patient's anatomy, increasing diagnostic utility.[57] However, since the scan obtained is primarily for localization purposes and not for detailed diagnostic imaging, low-dose CT for a PET/CT is sufficient.[58] Although generally covered by medical insurance when deemed medically necessary, many policies limit PET/CT scan coverage to the diagnostic work up and the first restaging scan 3 months after therapy completion.[59] Additionally, facilities incur steep fixed operational expenses associated with radiotracers, scanners, and maintenance, thus making them expensive for both patient and facility alike.[60,61]

PET/CT has excellent detection rate of primary tumors in the setting of SCC, with sensitivities of 94% and 97% for OPSCC and HNSCC, respectively.[62,63] MRI and CT are preferred in the pre-operative evaluation of submucosal extent and invasion of adjacent structures given their superior spatial resolution.[12,24] Thus, despite its accuracy in primary disease detection, PET/CT is restrained by a 4 to 5 mm resolution limit in current scanners, leading to a lack of anatomic detail that makes it unsuitable for the evaluation of these features.[64,65] Additionally, standard uptake value (SUV) measurements can be influenced by multiple factors. A systematic review by Adams and colleagues summarized the biologic and technical limitations in FDG distribution, including body size, blood glucose levels, scanner variability, image reconstruction parameters, among others, emphasizing the control of these to optimize SUV readings in the assessment of changes in metabolic activity.[66]

The NCCN Guidelines recommend using FDG-PET/CT for both nodal and distant metastases given its high specificity in detecting FDG-avid lesions.[21] For cervical lymph node assessment in patients with HNSCC, PET/CT is 81% sensitive and 98% specific, while providing a 95% diagnostic accuracy.[67] PET, with or without CT, has a sensitivity and specificity of 86% and 82%, respectively, for detection of residual or recurrent disease at the primary site.[68] It provides high sensitivity and specificity, 96% and 87% respectively, in detecting subclinical HNSCC recurrences 6 months after treatment completion.[69] Sensitivities and specificities for residual or recurrent neck disease were 72% and 88%, while for distant metastases these were 85% and 95%, respectively.[68] In the clinically N0 (cN0) neck, FDG-PET/CT has a sensitivity of 58% and specificity of 87%.[70] Also, for the cN0 neck, its negative predictive value is 87% as found by the ACRIN 6685 Trial.[71] HNC patients with tumors in the oral cavity, oropharynx, and supraglottic larynx benefit significantly from PET/CT, as these subsites have high rates of occult lymph node metastases.[72] Emerging literature also suggests that it is useful in detection of CUP in the setting of a biopsy-proven lymph node SCC.[73–75] PET/CT is preferred to panendoscopy when detecting synchronous primaries of the upper aerodigestive tract in the setting of HNSCC, where it reveals concurrent lesions with 100% sensitivity and 96% specificity.[76,77]

Despite the advantages brought forth by FDG-PET/CT, detection of microscopic disease remains elusive. Physiologic FDG uptake in the H&N is seen in multiple structures, including Waldeyer's ring and muscles in the larynx and pharynx.[78] There are many potential pitfalls in H&N PET/CT imaging, including inflammatory uptake in lymph nodes, uptake in brown fat, as well as asymmetric physiologic uptake within the tonsillar lymphoid tissue and larynx.[79] Additionally, benign etiologies such as Warthin's tumors and oncocytomas of the salivary glands have increased uptake due to increased mitochondrial content.[80] Inflammatory changes after treatment or biopsy also lead to increased FDG-avidity which can make post-treatment surveillance imaging with PET/CT challenging (**Fig. 3**).[81–83]

However, PET/CT is no longer the sole hybrid imaging modality, as PET/MRI is one of the newer modalities available for clinical use. This technology makes use of the functional metabolic aspect of target tissues identified by PET imaging while leveraging the detailed soft tissue contrast on MRI scans.[84] A clear advantage PET/MRI has over conventional PET/CT is the absence of ionizing radiation exposure, especially relevant in patients undergoing multiple scans for staging of primary disease and restaging after treatment.[85] Additionally, PET/MRI capitalizes on (1) the contrast offered by MRI sequences, such as diffusion-weighted imaging (DWI), (2) gives available time to collect PET data, and (3) allows for better motion correction compared to PET/CT.[86] In line with MRI technology, PET/MRI has an added time cost to multiple-bed-position PET, although the clinical applications in which PET/MRI provides an advantage over PET/CT may require a single bed position.[87,88] Furthermore, the high resolution of MRI is asymmetrically matched to the very low resolution of the PET-based imaging agents, making it impractical for preoperative planning.

A review of PET/MRI in oncology by Morsing and colleagues describes applications in HNC.[89] PET/MRI is superior to PET/CT in primary tumor extent assessment in nasopharyngeal cancer, where it correctly identified invasion of the pterygopalatine fossa, intracranial extension, and perineural infiltration in 5, 11, and 14 patients additional patients compared to PET/CT.[90] Although it demonstrated superior detection of regional lymph nodes, with a sensitivity of 99.5% compared to 91% on PET/CT for N staging, this difference was not statistically different for their cohort.[90] Studies by Kubiessa and colleagues and Schaarschmidt and colleagues found no differences in tumor staging for HNSCC with PET/MRI compared to PET/CT, where it revealed a sensitivity of 81% and specificity of 88% in primary tumor detection in the former and a diagnostic accuracy of 75% and 71% for T and N stage, respectively, in the latter.[91,92] Because metabolism of glucose is highly sensitive but less specific, there has been a focus on use of novel tumor-specific agents such as prostate-specific membrane antigen (PSMA) for imaging of salivary gland malignancies (see below).

Ultrasound

US utilizes high-energy, ultrasonic (above the audible range for humans—20 kHz) sound waves to detect structures by bouncing off these, creating images derived

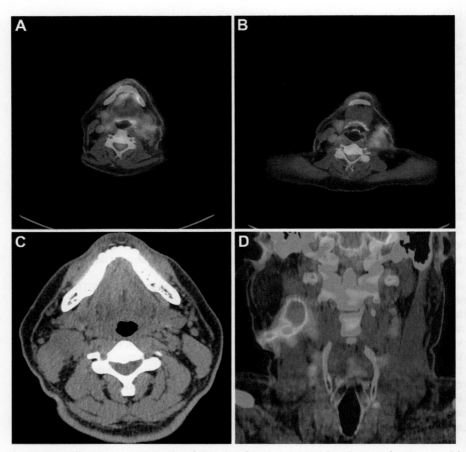

Fig. 3. Cases illustrating potential pitfalls in performing PET/CT. (*A, B*) Case of a 77-year-old male who underwent PET/CT imaging 2 weeks after left side neck dissection. (*C, D*) Case of a 38-year-old male who underwent an US-guided needle biopsy of a necrotic, fluid-filled level II node followed by PET/CT imaging 4 hours later. PET/CT fusion image showed localized metabolic activity along the needle's trajectory. Both of these cases highlight the challenges presented by utilizing PET/CT prematurely following an intervention.

from the "echo" of the waves that are reflected to the probe.[93] Wave propagation characteristics, such as speed and reflection, depend on the media they are traveling through, thus limiting transmission by bone and air.[94] These 2 possess high and low acoustic impedances, respectively, resulting in high reflection of waves in the former and scattering of US waves in the latter.[93,95] Unlike CT and MRI, ultrasound provides real-time dynamic assessments without any risk associated with radiation exposure, providing reliable, quick, accessible, and inexpensive imaging.[96–98] In patients with OCSCC, US can be used for primary tumor assessment, lymph node status, staging, and post-treatment surveillance.[99,100] Intraoperatively, US can provide real-time tumor measurements, margin assessment, and guided neck dissections.[101] Its application remains limited by operator experience and poor definition of deep anatomic structures, such as the retropharyngeal nodes.[24,97]

Using US to evaluate H&N swellings and masses after clinical evaluation was found to offer both sensitivity and specificity of 100% compared to clinical diagnosis alone.[96] Though it is not a modality of choice in initial workup and evaluation of HNC, it can be superior to traditional modalities like MRI in capturing tumor thickness and tumors that are smaller in size.[101] It has been noted to offer superior insight into depth of invasion for patients with T1-2 oral tongue SCC compared to MRI.[102]

When considering investigation of a primary tumor, US is most commonly used in the work up of thyroid cancer, in accordance with the NCCN Clinical Practice Guidelines in Oncology for Thyroid Carcinoma Version 1.2024.[103] Fine-needle aspiration (FNA) with ultrasound guidance is the procedure of choice for evaluating suspicious thyroid nodules.[104,105] However, several guidelines exist in using sonographic characteristics to assess the need for FNA, allowing for minimally invasive diagnostic evaluations without further biopsy.[105,106]

Nodal status frequently serves as an important prognostic indicator in HNC.[107] US has the ability to identify and accurately stage lymph node metastasis. By informing on vascular patterns of cervical lymph nodes, Doppler sonography US can aid in identification of benign versus malignant nodes.[108,109] In HNSCC, US-guided FNA has been documented to provide more accurate nodal cytology for N staging preoperatively than palpation, MRI, CT, or US alone (69%, 82%, 78%, 75%, respectively, vs 90% in US-guided FNA) with similar trends noted in sensitivity (67%, 82%, 83%, 75% vs 90%) and specificity (73%, 81%, 70%, 75% vs 100%).[110] Compared to FNA, US has a sensitivity of 75% and specificity of 86% in detecting metastatic nodes in patients with OCSCC.[111] US-guided FNA biopsy shows significantly improved sensitivity when compared to palpation-guided FNA in identifying nodal metastasis (48% vs 83%).[112]

US is particularly useful in the initial evaluation of H&N masses in the pediatric population, as it can be done with relatively little discomfort, without sedation, and eliminates radiation exposure concerns.[113] In addition to distinguishing between cystic and solid masses, advancements in high-resolution grey-scale US, including Doppler imaging, is very beneficial when considering vascular malformations in the pediatric population.[114]

Current Imaging Guidelines

Current NCCN guidelines for HNC (V.2.2024) recommend using CT or MRI for the initial workup for primary tumor assessment.[21] Generally, CT is performed as the initial modality, although MRI is preferred when there is suspicion of bone marrow involvement, orbital or skull base invasion, perineural tumor spread, or extensive dental amalgam. Primary site imaging with CT or MRI should include the anatomy from the skull base to the thoracic inlet to include any nodal disease. In the setting of CUP, PET/CT is recommended before evaluation under anesthesia, biopsy, or tonsillectomy. Image-guided (US or CT) FNA can provide further diagnostic information. Nodal metastasis is typically evaluated using CT or MRI during primary site imaging but may include chest CT or FDG-PET/CT, especially the latter if the tumor encroaches on the midline or definitive RT is warranted. For patients with locoregionally advanced disease (T3-4 primary or ≥N1 nodal stage), FDG-PET/CT is preferred except where brain metastases are suspected in which contrast-enhanced brain MRI should be obtained. Chest CT may be used to assess pulmonary metastases and mediastinal adenopathy if FDG-PET/CT is not performed. Additional imaging with CT or MRI during the short-term post-operative period is recommended for patients with locoregionally advanced disease, those with signs of early recurrence, and for cases where incomplete response is a concern. FDG-PET/CT should be performed 3 to 6 months after therapeutic course completion due to its high sensitivity.[68,115] FDG-PET/CT scans should not be performed within 12 weeks of systemic treatment or radiotherapy due to high false-positive rates.[78]

NEW TECHNIQUES FOR HEAD AND NECK CANCER IMAGING
Molecular Imaging

The visualization and quantification of biochemical activity *in vivo* has the potential to unmask the clinical biology of HNC and can be achieved through molecular imaging.[116,117] Tumor assessment through this lens opens the door to a myriad of possibilities in oncological management, including diagnosis, staging, therapeutic target assessment, and monitoring therapeutic response.[117] There are numerous modalities currently available, including intraoperative optical imaging with fluorescent probes, novel radiotracers for PET scans, functional MRI, and single-photon emission CT (SPECT).[116,118,119]

Similar to glucose radiotracers, thymidine radiotracers exploit cell-trapping mechanisms that further polarize the molecule and render it uncapable of leaving the cell.[120] As opposed to other nucleosides, thymidine only incorporates into DNA molecules.[121] Several studies have established the role of 3'-deoxy-3'-(^{18}F)-fluorothymidine PET (^{18}F-FLT PET) as a reliable marker for DNA synthesis and tumor cell proliferation, including a meta-analysis that found significant correlation between ^{18}F-FLT and Ki-67 across 27 studies.[122–124] Thymidine radiotracers may circumvent limitations posed by ^{18}F-FDG-PET, as there is little physiologic uptake within the body and thus may aid in assessing response to treatment.[125–127] Troost and colleagues reported ^{18}F-FLT-PET/CT signal changes precede volumetric tumor response during RT for both oropharyngeal primary tumors and metastatic lymph nodes.[128] For patients undergoing RT for HNSCC, Kishino and colleagues suggest ^{18}F-FLT uptake, compared to ^{18}F-FDG, may have improved specificity for early locoregional outcomes during (72% vs 19%, respectively) and after (80% vs 48%) RT.[129] Similar trends were reported for overall accuracy during (74% vs 30%, for ^{18}F-FLT and ^{18}F-FDG, respectively) and after (81% vs 57%) therapy.[129] In addition, Hoeben and colleagues found that changes in ^{18}F-FLT-PET/CT uptake early during RT or chemoradiotherapy (CRT) is a strong predictor for oncologic outcomes, with large decreases in uptake during the second week of treatment predicting more favorable outcomes.[130] Taken together, results from these studies suggest that ^{18}F-FLT-PET has the potential to significantly impact HNC care, allowing for treatment to be modified based on biologic response to therapy.

Hypoxia

Hypoxia within the tumor microenvironment has been shown to drive epigenetic modifications that set the stage for tumor angiogenesis and vasculogenesis, leading to epithelial-mesenchymal transition and ultimately potentiating metastases.[131–133] These features are known to precede tumor survival, growth, and invasiveness, leading to an immunosuppressive environment that amplifies resistance to therapy.[131] Briefly, immunosuppressive regulatory T-cells and myeloid-derived suppressor cells infiltrate hypoxic tumors, suppressing cytotoxic T-cells and decreasing immune surveillance through tumor growth factor-β, IL-10, and vascular endothelial growth factor expression.[134–136] HNSCC are amongst the most hypoxic tumors and thus promote expression of these immunosuppressive markers.[137] Hypoxic environments confer resistance to RT by cutting off the supply of the effector molecules in RT: reactive oxygen species (ROS).[138] Aerobic conditions allow ROS to wreak havoc in tumor tissues, overwhelming cellular DNA repair mechanisms and contributing to cell death.[139] Thus, development of tools that improve intratumoral hypoxic environment assessment is necessary.

[18]F-fluoromisonidazole PET (^{18}F-FMISO PET) has been identified as a potentially reliable imaging method for non-invasive monitoring of tumor hypoxia.[140–142] Patients with persistent tumor hypoxia on ^{18}F-FMISO PET and high programmed death-ligand 1 expression on tumor cells exhibit inferior outcomes compared to those with early hypoxia responses.[143] Patients with both tumor and lymph node hypoxia have been found to have inferior outcomes compared to those with tumor-only hypoxia.[143,144] Patients with locally advanced HNSCC can be stratified by hypoxic tumor volume on with ^{18}F-FMISO PET before CRT and 2 weeks into treatment.[145] Although with less success compared to ^{18}F-FMISO, similar nitroimidazole tracers, such as 2-(2-nitro-1H-imidazole-1-yl)-N-(2,2,3,3,3-penta-fluoropropyl)-acetamide (^{18}F-EF5), ^{18}F-fluoroerythronitromidazole (^{18}F-FETNIM), ^{18}F-fluoroazomycin-arabinofuranoside (^{18}F-FAZA), and ^{18}F-flortanidazole (^{18}F-HX4), have been investigated as a marker of hypoxia and consequently for response to radiation-based therapy.[146]

Multiple studies have examined Zirconiuim-89 ([89]Zr) as a radiotracer for antibody coupling, mainly due to its long half-life, *in vivo* stability, and physical characteristics.[147–151] Coupled with the anti-epidermal growth factor receptor (EGFR) antibody panitumumab for PET/CT scans ([89]Zr-pan PET/CT), this radiotracer exhibits minimally improved specificity for the detection of metastatic lymph nodes in HNSCC compared to ^{18}F-FDG PET/CT and improves the detection of HNSCC when combined with the latter.[152] A previous study by Börjesson and colleagues coupling [89]Zr to a CD44v6-targetted monoclonal antibody underpins its potential as a radioactive isotope in HNC detection.[153]

Margin assessment

Positive margins following oncologic H&N surgery lead to poor oncologic outcomes, and therefore have spurred investigation into technologies that may aid the surgeon in ensuring margin negativity.[154] Intraoperative molecular imaging may enable localization and identification of disease that cannot be detected by white light, and thus aids in achieving a complete resection intraoperatively.[155–157] Current imaging techniques used to improve surgical margins include narrow-band imaging, frozen section analysis, and ultrasound.[158] Yet, positive margin rates in the HNC remain suboptimal.[159] In HNSCC, the use of anti-EGFR-targeted agents with fluorescent labels (panitumumab-IRDye800CW) has the potential to detect clear differentiation between tumor and normal tissue while predicting distance of tumor tissue to specimen surface on the basis of fluorescence intensity.[160,161] Additional studies have shown a potential role for panitumumab-IRDye800CW in lymph node mapping in patients undergoing elective neck dissection for HNC.[162,163] Cetuximab-800CW, also an EGFR-targeted antibody, shows promising diagnostic accuracy for intraoperative surgical margin adjustment and postoperative lymph node examination in OCSCC.[164,165] Ongoing trials in the field are investigating the use of pH-sensitive micellar polymer (pegsitacianine) that release indocyanine green (ICG) in low pH tumor microenvironment and can detect positive margins and occult disease.[166]

Prostate-specific membrane antigen

Research exploring PSMA, a transmembrane glycoprotein of the prostate secretory acinar epithelium that is upregulated in prostate cancer, suggests it is an important immunohistological marker involved in tumor angiogenesis.[167–169] In the H&N, studies have focused on investigating increased PSMA expression among minor salivary gland tumors, especially in adenoid cystic carcinoma (ACC), and have suggested the potential for PSMA-targeted imaging in staging and diagnosis (**Fig. 4**).[170–173] Additionally, it has the ability to detect metastatic brain lesions that are otherwise not picked up on standard FDG-PET/CT imaging.[174,175] This feature makes PSMA-PET a suitable diagnostic modality for imaging ACC of the minor salivary glands, where late presentation of distant metastatic disease affects more than a third of individuals 10+ years after treatment completion.[176,177] PSMA PET has also been studied in the identification of residual or recurrent disease in patients with juvenile nasopharyngeal angiofibroma.[178–181] Detection of these may have significant implications in targeted radiation treatment and may lead to improved quality of life.

Lymph Node Mapping

Lymph node involvement is often a key prognostic factor in cancer survival, staging, and treatment planning.[182–185] Therefore, identifying diseased nodes and sentinel lymph nodes (SLN) is an important consideration in the treatment of HNC. Among early-stage disease, many occult cervical metastases remain undetectable by current imaging techniques, including CT, MRI, PET/CT, and US.[186] Rudningen and colleagues suggest that while contrast-enhanced CT has some utility in ruling out nodal metastasis, the false-positive rate remains high.[187] Lymphatic drainage in the H&N region is complex and may be unpredictable, potentially decreasing the effectiveness of elective neck dissections.[186,188,189] For example, an oral tongue SCC may be treated with a partial glossectomy, and elective ipsilateral level I to IV neck dissection based on depth of invasion in a cN0 neck. While this is historically the correct treatment, if the lymphatic drainage from the tumor in fact drains to a node in the contralateral neck, the patient may receive unnecessary treatment to the ipsilateral neck and undertreatment of the contralateral neck.

Lymphoscintigraphy (LSG) has now been adopted in several disease sites to enable surgeons to investigate the primary lymph node(s) which drain a tumor basin, or the SLN.[190,191] The goal of this technique is to identify the correct node that is most likely

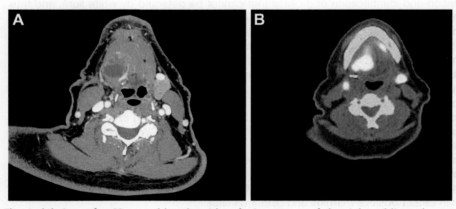

Fig. 4. (A) Case of a 68-year-old male with soft tissue mass of the right sublingual space invading the tongue and abutting the right mandible. Excisional biopsy showed adenocarcinoma, initially thought to be metastatic disease from prostate cancer primary. However, evaluation of Gleason score did not elucidate the diagnosis and a prostate-specific membrane antigen (PSMA) PET/CT was ordered. (A, B) PSMA PET/CT revealed marked radiotracer uptake at the right lateral aspect of the tongue and 2 lymph nodes, one in each level IIA and III, respectively. Surgical pathology revealed primary mucinous adenocarcinoma of the right sublingual gland with multiple (2) neck metastases.

involved with micro metastatic disease, and if none is found, limit the extent of neck dissection in order to minimize morbidity to the patient. In this technique, a radiotracer and/or visible dye is injected around the tumor and traced using imaging techniques to identify the SLN.[192,193] The most common radiotracer used is ^{99m}Tc-labeled sulfur colloid, although nanocolloid or antimony trisulfide has also been used.[188] Prior to surgery, the patient receives peritumoral injections with the radiotracer and imaging is performed using a gamma camera to identify the SLN basin.[193,194]

Following imaging identification of SLN location, in the operating room, the surgeon will then usually inject a second visible tracer, such as methylene blue or isosulfan blue, prior to incision.[188] Once in the region of the SLN, the surgeon will commonly use an intraoperative handheld gamma probe to identify the area of high activity and may confirm the sentinel lymph node biopsy (SLNB) by identifying visible tracer accumulation within the SLN.[195] Overall, a meta-analysis by Liu and colleagues found this technique to have an SLN identification rate of 96%, a sensitivity of 87%, and a 94% negative predictive value.[196]

Hybrid imaging with SPECT and CT (SPECT/CT) is an active area of exploration that provides complementary scintigraph and morphologic data regarding localization of the SLN.[197] Although SPECT/CT improves localization over conventional planar imaging, SPECT has a resolution of 8 to 12 mm (compared to 4–6 mm for PET) and higher radiation exposure compared to PET. In a prospective trial, NCT02572661, it was established that SLN metastases could define the extent of RT in patients with HNSCC, suggesting the use of lymph node mapping with SPECT/CT[198] These findings have sparked interest in exploring the use of SPECT/CT to tailor treatment plans among HNC patients.[199,200] Additionally, a separate phase III randomized trial by the Canadian Cancer Trails Group, CCTG-HN11, is studying the use of an SPECT/CT lymphatic mapping approach to RT of the contralateral neck.[201]

While now part of standard practice of recommendation for cutaneous malignancies such as melanoma and SCC, SLNB is being investigated in oral cavity and oropharynx malignancies.[202] SLNB and subsequent dissection utilizing lymphatic drainage mapping has been recommended as an alternative to elective neck dissection in early OCSCC.[203] One of the primary early concerns with this application was the "shine through effect" where the primary tumor gamma radiation would obscure adjacent SLN.[204] However, with improved techniques and options, such as 3D SPECT/CT, this may be less of a concern (**Fig. 5**).[205,206] The utility of SLNB in early OCSCC is currently being studied by the NRG-HN006 trial.[207] A few studies have recently suggested similar applications for OPSCC.[183,198]

Additional non-invasive molecular imaging techniques have been applied in identification of metastatic lymph nodes.[208] Fluorescence molecular imaging using both conventional modalities, such as near-infrared (NIR), and novel materials, including various dyes and cellular compounds, can provide enhanced detection of lymph node metastases.[209,210] Several early-stage trials on NIR-I (700–900 nm) fluorescence imaging have identified various agents capable of rapidly identifying metastatic nodes and tumor tissue in real time, namely OLT38, LUM015, and bevacizumab-IRDye800CW.[211,212] Krishnan and colleagues found that panitumumab-IRDye800CW preferentially localized to metastatic and SLNs in patients with OCSCC when delivered intravenously during the preoperative period.[163] Although pending final results, a subsequent clinical trial, NCT03733210, has recently completed assessing the ability of ^{89}Zr-panitumumab and ^{18}F-FDG to detect lymph node disease in patients with HNSCC.[213] The ongoing investigation and development of these techniques hold tremendous value and potential to improve diagnostic accuracy and early detection of lymphatic metastases.

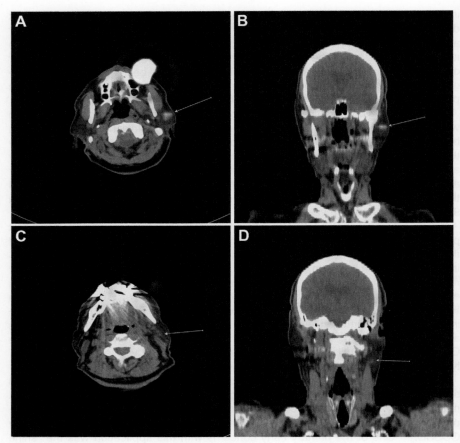

Fig. 5. Case of an 83-year-old male presenting with a merkel cell carcinoma of the left lower eyelid. Prior to undergoing wide-local excision, the patient underwent lymphoscintigraphy with single-photon emission computed tomography/CT for preoperative planning of sentinel lymph node biopsy. (*A, B*) Imaging revealed increased tracer activity (*yellow arrows*) at the superior margin of the superficial left parotid gland in the preauricular region. (*C, D*) Tracer activity (*yellow arrows*) was also detected immediately superficial to the upper left sternocleidomastoid muscle.

Novel Endoscopic Techniques

While CT and MRI are often used to detect submucosal spread and extent of disease, they may fail to detect smaller superficial mucosal lesions.[214] Developments in endoscopic techniques and imaging may allow for detection and diagnosis of early stage OCSCC.[215–217] Narrow band imaging (NBI) is among one of the most widely available endoscopic imaging methods.[218] The potential use of NBI in screening and diagnosis of HNCs has been previously explored.[219–223] It serves to highlight increased vascularity and neoangiogenesis without the use of dyes by filtering standard white light into 2 wavelengths.[219,224] It has been noted to improve the screening and surveillance of H&N lesions, particularly in the oropharynx and hypopharynx, during routine endoscopic examination when compared to standard imaging.[222,225] NBI can provide better detection of irregular vascular patterns and better visualization when compared to conventional laryngoscopy.[226] In conjunction with magnifying endoscopy, it may be used to accurately detect superficial SCCs and determine lesion extent, optimal surgical margins, and radiation fields in patients with advanced oropharyngeal and hypopharyngeal cancer.[227,228] The technique has also been applied intraoperatively to aid in intraoperative tissue biopsy.[229] However, a study noted that among tonsillar SCC, autofluorescence was superior in determining endoscopic signs of tumor spread and malignancy.[230] This technology may improve the screening and surveillance of H&N lesions during routine endoscopic examination when compared to standard imaging.[222,225] Among individuals with prior RT, ulcers, or infections, the false-positive rate can be high.[231–233]

Also utilized in assessing OCSCC endoscopically, autofluorescence imaging allows for visualization and assessment of tumor extent and has been investigated in HNC.[234–236] It uses exogenous fluorescent tracers that target cancer cells to identify and assess tumor tissue.[160,237] The presence of several endogenous fluorophores results in tumor tissue fluorescence changes, and consequently, their lifetime of fluorescence.[238] These changes can be measured to varying sensitivities depending on the florescent agent used.[234] In comparison to NBI, it may be more accurate in identifying irregular tissue and mucosal margins and may also be able to determine the depth of tumor.[236] Among the oldest clinically available agents is ICG. This agent is largely untargeted and relies on perfusion and accumulation in tumor tissue due to enhanced permeability and retention in neoplastic tissue as a result of disrupted tumor neovasculature.[239] A review by De Ravin and colleagues noted ICG had a pooled sensitivity and specificity of 92% and 72%, respectively, in assessing tumor margins.[240]

NIR using ICG is often used for SLN identification intraoperatively although its application is largely limited by the rapid clearance of these fluorophores.[241] 5-aminolevulinic acid (5-ALA) is another agent utilized in fluorescence imaging that provides more tumor-specific affinity, though this has extensively been studied in gliomas.[242] Due to unspecific binding, ICG can accumulate in peritumoral edema, leading to hindered specificity and false positivity.[243] 5-ALA offers tumor-specific fluorescence due to the accumulation of its fluorogenic metabolite, protoporphyrin IX, in tumor tissue.[242] Still, it has been established to successfully detect HNC.[244,245] One study noted a specificity of 60% and a sensitivity of 99% when assessing OCSCC.[245] In a separate study, 5-ALA was reported to be useful intraoperatively to predict perineural invasion, positive margins, and metastatic lymphadenopathy in HNC.[246]

Radiomics and Artificial Intelligence

Radiomics is an emerging field in medical imaging that involves extracting a large number of quantitative features from medical images using data-characterization algorithms.[247] Briefly, it seeks to identify patterns in large datasets, improve accuracy compared to the naked eye, and associate outcomes based on pattern recognition and diagnosis. This has the potential to enhance diagnostic, prognostic, and predictive accuracy in oncology and influence the era of personalized medicine.[248] In the oral cavity, radiomic signatures have been found to outperform clinical and pathologic TNM stages as prognostic signatures and allowed investigators to correctly predict survival outcomes.[249,250]

A systematic review found radiomics-based analyses to be potentially helpful in predicting occult lymph node metastases for patients with OCSCC.[251] For oropharyngeal tumors, radiomics research shows promise in predicting HPV status, prognosis, recurrence, and overall survival for OPSCC.[252–258] Kowalchuck and colleagues proposed to stratify patients with HPV(+)OPSCC for treatment de-escalation on the basis of radiologic N stage, where patients with up to 4 involved lymph nodes (rN0-1) had a 93% to 94% chance of remaining pN0-1.[259] Peritumoral and intratumoral radiomic models have potential for predicting overall survival and progression-free survival in patients undergoing definitive RT for laryngeal and hypopharyngeal cancer.[260] Similarly, relevant models may be able to identify treatment-sensitive tumors in HNC patients who may benefit from selected therapies.[261] For example, a radiomic model established by Lu and colleagues risk-stratified patients with HNSCC into low, medium, or high risk for platinum-refractory disease based on MRI texture features.[262] In a similar fashion, MRI-based radiomic features demonstrate an area under the curve of 0.85 and an accuracy of 81% in predicting tumor-infiltrating lymphocyte levels in patients with oral tongue SCC, potentially leading to risk-stratification for immunotherapeutic agents in immuno-sensitive tumors.[263,264]

Artificial intelligence (AI) encompasses a wide range of capabilities, including reasoning and problem-solving. The evolution of computational power has enabled unprecedented research of digital images and has allowed the integration of radiomic, clinical, and genomic datasets. AI algorithms can achieve a high degree of accuracy to aid in HNC detection that may exceed the abilities of human judgment in data prediction.[265]

Additionally, machine learning (ML) has the capacity to enhance radiomic analysis by identifying complex patterns within radiomic features and uncover new characteristics not initially identified. For example, ML models trained on metabolic parameters derived from ^{18}F-FDG PET/CT outperform models using PET/CT or clinical parameters alone when classifying HPV status in OPSCC.[266] Texture analysis of dual-energy CT (DECT) images assisted by ML can help distinguish neoplastic from inflammatory nodes on top of correctly identifying normal from pathologic lymph nodes.[267] A deep learning algorithm reported by Klein and colleagues was able to determine HPV status from hematoxylin & eosin histologic slides accurately, outperforming gold-standard HPV testing with p16 or HPV-DNA.[268] Beyond diagnostic, prognostic, and risk-stratification applications, deep-learning algorithms seem well equipped to aid the radiation oncologist in RT planning as outlined by Bibault and Giraud.[269] From the authors' review of the literature, it is evident that research into future applications for AI within HNC is critical. A recent survey study by Chen and colleagues revealed increased physician trust in ML clinical decision support tools among otolaryngologists, supporting the observed heightened interests in AI research for HNC.[270]

FUTURE DIRECTIONS

The exploration of novel imaging techniques for HNC highlights several promising avenues. Improving understanding of the biology of HNC has enabled research of multiple biochemical agents that have augmented or inspired novel imaging modalities. Interdisciplinary collaborations across the scientific community, blending insights from medical physics, radiology, computer science, electrical, mechanical, and biomedical engineering, among other fields, have paved the way for innovative approaches to enhanced HNC detection, staging, surveillance, and will hopefully contribute to improved outcomes. However, there is a need to address the gap between emerging trends in cancer diagnosis and imaging modalities poised to supplement, not complicate diagnostic guidelines and recommendations.

Current imaging techniques, including those novel imaging technologies reviewed earlier, still fall short of the needs of our patients. We currently have no reliable tumor-specific imaging techniques and are limited by the size of detectable disease, physiologic normal tissue attributes, and innumerable technique limitations. With the introduction of MCED tests that will routinely identify patients with HNC often before a tumor is clinically detectable, improved resolution will become even more critical. In the HPV era, overcoming the confounding impact of FDG avidity within normal tonsil tissue will be critical in identifying microscopic or sub centimeter tumors and allowing for early intervention.

SUMMARY

While CT, MRI, PET/CT, and US remain the foundational imaging for HNC, novel technologies have the potential to augment and, in some cases, replace these traditional techniques. It is incumbent on the H&N oncologist to be aware of not only the advantages and limitations of the core techniques but also of the potential to utilize novel opportunities. Further research is needed into biology-driven imaging technology and all techniques and their interpretations will likely be augmented by AI and ML in the very near future. Clinicians and investigators should remain aware of the impact these advances will have on our patients.

CLINICS CARE POINTS

- Squamous cell carcinoma accounts for over 90% of all HNC.
- Imaging studies serve as the foundation for treatment decision making.
- CT and MRI are the modalities of choice for the assessment of tumor extent and regional invasion.
- PET/CT is very specific for the evaluation of nodal and distant metastases in HNSCC.
- Ultrasound is useful for the evaluatuion of nodal masses, especially with FNA guidance.
- Molecular imaging, lymph node mapping, and endoscopic techniques have the potential to augment conventional techniques.

DISCLOSURE

There are no relevant conflicts of interest to disclose.

REFERENCES

1. Chi AC, Day TA, Neville BW. Oral cavity and oropharyngeal squamous cell carcinoma–an update. CA Cancer J Clin 2015;65(5):401–21.
2. Naegele S, Ruiz-Torres DA, Zhao Y, et al. Comparing the Diagnostic Performance of Quantitative PCR, Digital Droplet PCR, and Next-Generation Sequencing Liquid Biopsies for Human Papillomavirus-Associated Cancers. J Mol Diagn 2023. https://doi.org/10.1016/j.jmoldx.2023.11.007.
3. Neal RD, Johnson P, Clarke CA, et al. Cell-Free DNA-Based Multi-Cancer Early Detection Test in an Asymptomatic Screening Population (NHS-Galleri): design of a pragmatic, prospective randomised controlled trial. Cancers 2022;14(19).
4. Nicholson BD, Oke J, Virdee PS, et al. Multi-cancer early detection test in symptomatic patients referred for cancer investigation in England and Wales (SYMPLIFY): a large-scale, observational cohort study. Lancet Oncol 2023;24(7): 733–43.

5. Schrag D, Beer TM, McDonnell CH, et al. Blood-based tests for multicancer early detection (PATHFINDER): a prospective cohort study. Lancet 2023; 402(10409):1251–60.

6. Rettig EM, Wang AA, Tran N-A, et al. Association of pretreatment circulating tumor tissue–modified viral HPV DNA with clinicopathologic factors in HPV-Positive Oropharyngeal Cancer. JAMA Otolaryngology–Head & Neck Surgery 2022;148(12):1120–30.

7. Batool S, Sethi RKV, Wang A, et al. Circulating tumor-tissue modified HPV DNA testing in the clinical evaluation of patients at risk for HPV-positive oropharynx cancer: The IDEA-HPV study. Oral Oncol 2023;147:106584.

8. Thawley SE, Gado M, Fuller TR. Computerized tomography in the evaluation of head and neck lesions. Laryngoscope 1978;88(3):451–9.

9. Uyl-de Groot CA, Senft A, de Bree R, et al. Chest CT and whole-body 18F-FDG PET are cost-effective in screening for distant metastases in head and neck cancer patients. J Nucl Med 2010;51(2):176–82.

10. Kurien G, Hu J, Harris J, et al. Cost-effectiveness of positron emission tomography/computed tomography in the management of advanced head and neck cancer. J Otolaryngol Head Neck Surg 2011;40(6):468–72.

11. Peh WCG. Pitfalls in diagnostic radiology. Springer 2015;x:543.

12. Cheung YK, Sham J, Cheung YL, et al. Evaluation of skull base erosion in nasopharyngeal carcinoma: comparison of plain radiography and computed tomography. Oncology Jan-Feb 1994;51(1):42–6.

13. Bae YJ, Kim TE, Choi BS, et al. Comprehensive assessments of the open mouth dynamic maneuver and metal artifact reduction algorithm on computed tomography images of the oral cavity and oropharynx. PLoS One 2021;16(3): e0248696.

14. Weissman JL, Carrau RL. "Puffed-cheek" CT improves evaluation of the oral cavity. AJNR Am J Neuroradiol 2001;22(4):741–4.

15. Di Martino E, Nowak B, Hassan HA, et al. Diagnosis and staging of head and neck cancer: a comparison of modern imaging modalities (positron emission tomography, computed tomography, color-coded duplex sonography) with pan-endoscopic and histopathologic findings. Arch Otolaryngol Head Neck Surg 2000;126(12):1457–61.

16. Shingaki S, Suzuki I, Nakajima T, et al. Computed tomographic evaluation of lymph node metastasis in head and neck carcinomas. J Cranio-Maxillofacial Surg 1995;23(4):233–7.

17. Stevens MH, Harnsberger HR, Mancuso AA, et al. Computed tomography of cervical lymph nodes: staging and management of head and neck cancer. Arch Otolaryngol 1985;111(11):735–9.

18. Taghipour M, Mena E, Kruse MJ, et al. Post-treatment 18F-FDG-PET/CT versus contrast-enhanced CT in patients with oropharyngeal squamous cell carcinoma: comparative effectiveness study. Nucl Med Commun 2017;38(3):250–8.

19. Amin MB, Edge SB, Greene FL, et al. AJCC cancer staging manual1024. Cham, Switzerland: Springer; 2017.

20. Sun J, Li B, Li CJ, et al. Computed tomography versus magnetic resonance imaging for diagnosing cervical lymph node metastasis of head and neck cancer: a systematic review and meta-analysis. OncoTargets Ther 2015;8:1291–313.

21. Referenced with permission from the NCCN Clinical Practice Guidelines in Oncology (NCCN Guidelines®) for Head and Neck Cancers V.2.2024. © National Comprehensive Cancer Network, Inc. All rights reserved. Accessed

January 19, 2024, To view the most recent and complete version of the guideline, go online to NCCN.org.

22. Duprez F, Berwouts D, De Neve W, et al. Distant metastases in head and neck cancer. Head Neck 2017;39(9):1733–43.

23. Pfister DG, Spencer S, Adelstein D, et al. Head and Neck Cancers, Version 2.2020, NCCN Clinical Practice Guidelines in Oncology. J Natl Compr Cancer Netw 2020;18(7):873–98.

24. Junn JC, Soderlund KA, Glastonbury CM. Imaging of Head and Neck Cancer With CT, MRI, and US. Semin Nucl Med 2021;51(1):3–12.

25. Abdullaeva U, Pape B, Hirvonen J. Diagnostic Accuracy of MRI in Detecting the Perineural Spread of Head and Neck Tumors: A Systematic Review and Meta-Analysis. Diagnostics 2024;14(1).

26. Choi HY, Yoon DY, Kim ES, et al. Diagnostic performance of CT, MRI, and their combined use for the assessment of the direct cranial or intracranial extension of malignant head and neck tumors. Acta Radiol 2019;60(3):301–7.

27. Handschel J, Naujoks C, Depprich RA, et al. CT-scan is a valuable tool to detect mandibular involvement in oral cancer patients. Oral Oncol 2012;48(4):361–6.

28. Glastonbury CM. Nasopharyngeal carcinoma: the role of magnetic resonance imaging in diagnosis, staging, treatment, and follow-up. Top Magn Reson Imag 2007;18(4):225–35.

29. Abd El-Hafez YG, Chen C-C, Ng S-H, et al. Comparison of PET/CT and MRI for the detection of bone marrow invasion in patients with squamous cell carcinoma of the oral cavity. Oral Oncol 2011;47(4):288–95.

30. Nemzek WR, Hecht S, Gandour-Edwards R, et al. Perineural spread of head and neck tumors: how accurate is MR imaging? AJNR Am J Neuroradiol 1998;19(4):701–6.

31. Cho SJ, Lee JH, Suh CH, et al. Comparison of diagnostic performance between CT and MRI for detection of cartilage invasion for primary tumor staging in patients with laryngo-hypopharyngeal cancer: a systematic review and meta-analysis. Eur Radiol 2020;30(7):3803–12.

32. King AD, Vlantis AC, Yuen TW, et al. Detection of Nasopharyngeal Carcinoma by MR Imaging: Diagnostic Accuracy of MRI Compared with Endoscopy and Endoscopic Biopsy Based on Long-Term Follow-Up. AJNR Am J Neuroradiol 2015;36(12):2380–5.

33. Qu J, Pan B, Su T, et al. T1 and T2 mapping for identifying malignant lymph nodes in head and neck squamous cell carcinoma. Cancer Imag 2023;23(1):125.

34. Liao LJ, Lo WC, Hsu WL, et al. Detection of cervical lymph node metastasis in head and neck cancer patients with clinically N0 neck-a meta-analysis comparing different imaging modalities. BMC Cancer 2012;12:236.

35. Machczyński P, Majchrzak E, Niewinski P, et al. A review of the 8th edition of the AJCC staging system for oropharyngeal cancer according to HPV status. Eur Arch Oto-Rhino-Laryngol 2020;277(9):2407–12.

36. Park SI, Guenette JP, Suh CH, et al. The diagnostic performance of CT and MRI for detecting extranodal extension in patients with head and neck squamous cell carcinoma: a systematic review and diagnostic meta-analysis. Eur Radiol 2021;31(4):2048–61.

37. Jumper JR, Fischbein NJ, Kaplan MJ, et al. The "small, dark tonsil" in patients presenting with metastatic cervical lymphadenopathy from an unknown primary. AJNR Am J Neuroradiol 2005;26(2):411–3.

38. Cinar F. Significance of asymptomatic tonsil asymmetry. Otolaryngol Head Neck Surg 2004;131(1):101–3.

39. Choi YJ, Lee JH, Kim HO, et al. Histogram analysis of apparent diffusion coefficients for occult tonsil cancer in patients with cervical nodal metastasis from an unknown primary site at presentation. Radiology 2016;278(1):146–55.
40. Lee JH, Ha EJ, Roh J, et al. Technical feasibility of radiomics signature analyses for improving detection of occult tonsillar cancer. Sci Rep 2021;11(1):192.
41. Marshall EL, Ginat DT, Sammet S. mr imaging artifacts in the head and neck region: pitfalls and solutions. Neuroimaging Clin N Am 2022;32(2):279–86.
42. Lam P, Au-Yeung KM, Cheng PW, et al. Correlating MRI and histologic tumor thickness in the assessment of oral tongue cancer. AJR Am J Roentgenol 2004;182(3):803–8.
43. Jung J, Cho NH, Kim J, et al. Significant invasion depth of early oral tongue cancer originated from the lateral border to predict regional metastases and prognosis. Int J Oral Maxillofac Surg 2009;38(6):653–60.
44. Hilabi BS, Alghamdi SA, Almanaa M. Impact of magnetic resonance imaging on healthcare in low- and middle-income Countries. Cureus 2023;15(4):e37698.
45. van Beek EJR, Kuhl C, Anzai Y, et al. Value of MRI in medicine: More than just another test? J Magn Reson Imag 2019;49(7):e14–25.
46. AdvaMed. Why patients deserve priority in global semiconductor chips shortage. Available at: https://www.advamed.org/2022/06/06/why-patients-deserve-priority-in-global-semiconductor-chips-shortage/. [Accessed 11 February 2024].
47. Bradley BM S. How is the semiconductor shortage affecting medtech?. Available at: https://www2.deloitte.com/us/en/blog/health-care-blog/2022/how-is-the-semiconductor-shortage-affecting-medtech.html. [Accessed 11 February 2024].
48. Mahesh M, Barker PB. The MRI Helium Crisis: Past and Future. J Am Coll Radiol 2016;13(12 Pt A):1536–7.
49. Muthupillai R, Lomas DJ, Rossman PJ, et al. Magnetic resonance elastography by direct visualization of propagating acoustic strain waves. Science 1995;269(5232):1854–7.
50. Manduca A, Oliphant TE, Dresner MA, et al. Magnetic resonance elastography: non-invasive mapping of tissue elasticity. Med Image Anal 2001;5(4):237–54.
51. Suresh S. Biomechanics and biophysics of cancer cells. Acta Biomater 2007;3(4):413–38.
52. Jung HN, Ryoo I, Suh S, et al. Evaluating the Elasticity of Metastatic Cervical Lymph Nodes in Head and Neck Squamous Cell Carcinoma Patients Using DWI-based Virtual MR Elastography. Magn Reson Med Sci 2024;23(1):49–55.
53. Liu KH, Bhatia K, Chu W, et al. Shear wave elastography–a new quantitative assessment of post-irradiation neck fibrosis. Ultraschall der Med 2015;36(4):348–54.
54. Flint PW, Francis HW, Haughey BH, et al. Seventh edition. Cummings otolaryngology: head and neck surgery, vol 1. Elsevier; 2021.
55. Budinger TF, Derenzo SE, Huesman RH. Instrumentation for positron emission tomography. Ann Neurol 1984/01/01 1984;15(S1):35–43.
56. Phelps ME. Positron emission tomography provides molecular imaging of biological processes. Proc Natl Acad Sci USA 2000/08/01 2000;97(16):9226–33.
57. Kluetz PG, Meltzer CC, Villemagne VL, et al. Combined PET/CT Imaging in Oncology: Impact on Patient Management. Clinical Positron Imaging 2000;3(6):223–30.
58. Colsher JG, Kiang H, Thibault JB, et al. Ultra low dose CT for attenuation correction in PET/CT. 2008 IEEE Nuclear Science Symposium Conference Record. 2008: 5506-5511.

59. Services CfMaM. Coverage of Positron Emission Tomography Scans. Available at: https://www.cms.gov/medicare-coverage-database/view/ncd.aspx?ncdid=331.

60. Berger M, Gould MK, Barnett PG. The cost of positron emission tomography in six United States Veterans Affairs hospitals and two academic medical centers. AJR Am J Roentgenol 2003;181(2):359–65.

61. Chuck A, Jacobs P, Logus JW, et al. Marginal cost of operating a positron emission tomography center in a regulatory environment. Int J Technol Assess Health Care. Fall 2005;21(4):442–51.

62. Roh JL, Yeo NK, Kim JS, et al. Utility of 2-[18F] fluoro-2-deoxy-D-glucose positron emission tomography and positron emission tomography/computed tomography imaging in the preoperative staging of head and neck squamous cell carcinoma. Oral Oncol 2007;43(9):887–93.

63. Kim MR, Roh JL, Kim JS, et al. Utility of 18F-fluorodeoxyglucose positron emission tomography in the preoperative staging of squamous cell carcinoma of the oropharynx. Eur J Surg Oncol 2007;33(5):633–8.

64. Erdi YE. Limits of tumor detectability in nuclear medicine and PET. Mol Imaging Radionucl Ther 2012;21(1):23–8.

65. Moses WW. Fundamental limits of spatial resolution in PET. Nucl Instrum Methods Phys Res Sect A Accel Spectrom Detect Assoc Equip 2011/08/21/2011;648:S236–40.

66. Adams MC, Turkington TG, Wilson JM, et al. A systematic review of the factors affecting accuracy of SUV measurements. AJR Am J Roentgenol 2010;195(2):310–20.

67. Yoon DY, Hwang HS, Chang SK, et al. CT, MR, US,18F-FDG PET/CT, and their combined use for the assessment of cervical lymph node metastases in squamous cell carcinoma of the head and neck. Eur Radiol 2009;19(3):634–42.

68. Cheung PK, Chin RY, Eslick GD. Detecting residual/recurrent head neck squamous cell carcinomas using PET or PET/CT: systematic review and meta-analysis. Otolaryngol Head Neck Surg 2016;154(3):421–32.

69. Robin P, Abgral R, Valette G, et al. Diagnostic performance of FDG PET/CT to detect subclinical HNSCC recurrence 6 months after the end of treatment. Eur J Nucl Med Mol Imag 2015/01/01 2015;42(1):72–8.

70. Kim SJ, Pak K, Kim K. Diagnostic accuracy of F-18 FDG PET or PET/CT for detection of lymph node metastasis in clinically node negative head and neck cancer patients; A systematic review and meta-analysis. Am J Otolaryngol 2019;40(2):297–305.

71. Lowe VJ, Duan F, Subramaniam RM, et al. Multicenter Trial of [18F]fluorodeoxyglucose Positron Emission Tomography/Computed Tomography Staging of Head and Neck Cancer and Negative Predictive Value and Surgical Impact in the N0 Neck: Results From ACRIN 6685. J Clin Oncol 2019;37(20):1704–12.

72. Goel R, Moore W, Sumer B, et al. Clinical practice in PET/CT for the management of head and neck squamous cell cancer. Article. Am J Roentgenol 2017;209(2):289–303.

73. Kwee TC, Kwee RM. Combined FDG-PET/CT for the detection of unknown primary tumors: systematic review and meta-analysis. Eur Radiol 2009;19(3):731–44.

74. Johansen J, Buus S, Loft A, et al. Prospective study of 18FDG-PET in the detection and management of patients with lymph node metastases to the neck from an unknown primary tumor. Results from the DAHANCA-13 study. Head Neck 2008;30(4):471–8.

75. Rusthoven KE, Koshy M, Paulino AC. The role of fluorodeoxyglucose positron emission tomography in cervical lymph node metastases from an unknown primary tumor. Cancer 2004;101(11):2641–9.

76. Strobel K, Haerle SK, Stoeckli SJ, et al. Head and neck squamous cell carcinoma (HNSCC)–detection of synchronous primaries with (18)F-FDG-PET/CT. Eur J Nucl Med Mol Imag 2009;36(6):919–27.

77. Haerle SK, Strobel K, Hany TF, et al. (18)F-FDG-PET/CT versus panendoscopy for the detection of synchronous second primary tumors in patients with head and neck squamous cell carcinoma. Head Neck 2010;32(3):319–25.

78. Yeh R, Amer A, Johnson JM, et al. Pearls and pitfalls of 18FDG-PET head and neck imaging. Neuroimaging Clinics of North America 2022;32(2):287–98.

79. Bhargava P, Rahman S, Wendt J. Atlas of confounding factors in head and neck PET/CT imaging. Clin Nucl Med 2011;36(5):e20–9.

80. Patel ND, Av Zante, Eisele DW, et al. Oncocytoma: the vanishing parotid mass. Am J Neuroradiol 2011.

81. Sagardoy T, Fernandez P, Ghafouri A, et al. Accuracy of 18FDG PET-CT for treatment evaluation 3 months after completion of chemoradiotherapy for head and neck squamous cell carcinoma: 2-year minimum follow-up. Article. Head and Neck 2016;38:E1271–6.

82. Mori M, Tsukuda M, Horiuchi C, et al. Efficacy of fluoro-2-deoxy-d-glucose positron emission tomography to evaluate responses to concurrent chemoradiotherapy for head and neck squamous cell carcinoma. Article. Auris Nasus Larynx 2011;38(6):724–9.

83. Sjövall J, Wahlberg P, Almquist H, et al. A prospective study of positron emission tomography for evaluation of neck node response 6 weeks after radiotherapy in patients with head and neck squamous cell carcinoma. Article. Head and Neck 2016;38:E473–9.

84. Zaidi H, Mawlawi O, Orton CG. Point/counterpoint. Simultaneous PET/MR will replace PET/CT as the molecular multimodality imaging platform of choice. Med Phys 2007;34(5):1525–8.

85. Brix G, Lechel U, Glatting G, et al. Radiation exposure of patients undergoing whole-body dual-modality 18F-FDG PET/CT examinations. J Nucl Med 2005; 46(4):608–13.

86. Ehman EC, Johnson GB, Villanueva-Meyer JE, et al. PET/MRI: Where might it replace PET/CT? J Magn Reson Imag 2017;46(5):1247–62.

87. Vandenberghe S, Marsden PK. PET-MRI: a review of challenges and solutions in the development of integrated multimodality imaging. Phys Med Biol 2015; 60(4):R115–54.

88. Currie GM, Kamvosoulis P, Bushong S. PET/MRI, Part 2: Technologic Principles. J Nucl Med Technol 2021;49(3):217–25.

89. Morsing A, Hildebrandt MG, Vilstrup MH, et al. Hybrid PET/MRI in major cancers: a scoping review. Eur J Nucl Med Mol Imag 2019;46(10):2138–51.

90. Chan SC, Yeh CH, Yen TC, et al. Clinical utility of simultaneous whole-body (18) F-FDG PET/MRI as a single-step imaging modality in the staging of primary nasopharyngeal carcinoma. Eur J Nucl Med Mol Imag 2018;45(8):1297–308.

91. Kubiessa K, Purz S, Gawlitza M, et al. Initial clinical results of simultaneous 18F-FDG PET/MRI in comparison to 18F-FDG PET/CT in patients with head and neck cancer. Eur J Nucl Med Mol Imag 2014;41(4):639–48.

92. Schaarschmidt BM, Heusch P, Buchbender C, et al. Locoregional tumour evaluation of squamous cell carcinoma in the head and neck area: a comparison

between MRI, PET/CT and integrated PET/MRI. Eur J Nucl Med Mol Imag 2016; 43(1):92–102.

93. Joshi PS, Pol J, Sudesh AS. Ultrasonography - A diagnostic modality for oral and maxillofacial diseases. Contemp Clin Dent 2014;5(3):345–51.

94. Aldrich JE. Basic physics of ultrasound imaging. Crit Care Med 2007;35(5 Suppl):S131–7.

95. Coltrera MD. Ultrasound physics in a nutshell. Otolaryngol Clin North Am 2010; 43(6):1149–59.

96. Chandak R, Degwekar S, Bhowte RR, et al. An evaluation of efficacy of ultrasonography in the diagnosis of head and neck swellings. Dentomaxillofacial Radiol 2011;40(4):213–21.

97. Tshering Vogel DW, Thoeny HC. Cross-sectional imaging in cancers of the head and neck: how we review and report. Cancer Imag 2016;16(1):20.

98. Bulbul MG, Tarabichi O, Parikh AS, et al. The utility of intra-oral ultrasound in improving deep margin clearance of oral tongue cancer resections. Oral Oncol 2021;122:105512.

99. Lo WC, Chang CM, Cheng PC, et al. The Applications and Potential Developments of Ultrasound in Oral Cancer Management. Technol Cancer Res Treat 2022;21. 15330338221133216.

100. Jiang H, Tan Q, He F, et al. Ultrasound in patients with treated head and neck carcinomas: A retrospective analysis for effectiveness of follow-up care. Medicine (Baltim) 2021;100(16):e25496.

101. Yesuratnam A, Wiesenfeld D, Tsui A, et al. Preoperative evaluation of oral tongue squamous cell carcinoma with intraoral ultrasound and magnetic resonance imaging-comparison with histopathological tumour thickness and accuracy in guiding patient management. Int J Oral Maxillofac Surg 2014;43(7):787–94.

102. Nilsson O, Knutsson J, Landström FJ, et al. Ultrasound accurately assesses depth of invasion in T1-T2 oral tongue cancer. Laryngoscope Investig Otolaryngol 2022;7(5):1448–55.

103. Referenced with permission from the NCCN Clinical Practice Guidelines in Oncology (NCCN Guidelines®) for Thyroid Carcinoma V.1.2024. © National Comprehensive Cancer Network, Inc. All rights reserved. Accessed January 23, 2024, To view the most recent and complete version of the guideline, go online to NCCN.org.

104. Ezzat S, Sarti DA, Cain DR, et al. Thyroid incidentalomas. Prevalence by palpation and ultrasonography. Arch Intern Med 1994;154(16):1838–40.

105. Haugen BR, Alexander EK, Bible KC, et al. 2015 American Thyroid Association Management Guidelines for Adult Patients with Thyroid Nodules and Differentiated Thyroid Cancer: The American Thyroid Association Guidelines Task Force on Thyroid Nodules and Differentiated Thyroid Cancer. Thyroid 2016;26(1):1–133.

106. Tessler FN, Middleton WD, Grant EG, et al. ACR Thyroid Imaging, Reporting and Data System (TI-RADS): White Paper of the ACR TI-RADS Committee. J Am Coll Radiol 2017;14(5):587–95.

107. Layland MK, Sessions DG, Lenox J. The influence of lymph node metastasis in the treatment of squamous cell carcinoma of the oral cavity, oropharynx, larynx, and hypopharynx: N0 versus N+. Laryngoscope 2005;115(4):629–39.

108. Sumi M, Ohki M, Nakamura T. Comparison of sonography and CT for differentiating benign from malignant cervical lymph nodes in patients with squamous cell carcinoma of the head and neck. AJR Am J Roentgenol 2001;176(4):1019–24.

109. Yonetsu K, Sumi M, Izumi M, et al. Contribution of doppler sonography blood flow information to the diagnosis of metastatic cervical nodes in patients with head and neck cancer: assessment in relation to anatomic levels of the neck. AJNR Am J Neuroradiol 2001;22(1):163–9.

110. van den Brekel MW, Castelijns JA, Stel HV, et al. Modern imaging techniques and ultrasound-guided aspiration cytology for the assessment of neck node metastases: a prospective comparative study. Eur Arch Oto-Rhino-Laryngol 1993; 250(1):11–7.

111. Aggarwal A, Daniel MJ, Srinivasan S, et al. Grayscale ultrasonography in the assessment of regional lymph nodes in oral cancer and its correlation with TNM staging and FNAC. J Indian Acad Oral Med Radiol 2011;23(2):104–7.

112. Haller TJ, Van Abel KM, Yin LX, et al. Ultrasound Guided Biopsy in Patients With HPV-Associated Oropharyngeal Squamous Cell Carcinoma. Laryngoscope 2022;132(12):2396–402.

113. Abramson ZR, Nagaraj UD, Lai LM, et al. Imaging of pediatric head and neck tumors: A COG Diagnostic Imaging Committee/SPR Oncology Committee/ASPNR White Paper. Pediatr Blood Cancer 2023;70(Suppl 4):e30151.

114. Imhof H, Czerny C, Hörmann M, et al. Tumors and tumor-like lesions of the neck: from childhood to adult. Eur Radiol Suppl 2004;14(4):L155–65.

115. Heineman TE, Kuan EC, St John MA. When should surveillance imaging be performed after treatment for head and neck cancer? Laryngoscope 2017;127(3):533–4.

116. Wu J, Yuan Y, Tao XF. Targeted molecular imaging of head and neck squamous cell carcinoma: a window into precision medicine. Chin Med J (Engl) 2020;133(11):1325–36.

117. Mankoff DA. A definition of molecular imaging. J Nucl Med 2007;48(6):18n–21n.

118. Pysz MA, Gambhir SS, Willmann JK. Molecular imaging: current status and emerging strategies. Clin Radiol 2010;65(7):500–16.

119. Shah D, Gehani A, Mahajan A, et al. Advanced Techniques in Head and Neck Cancer Imaging: Guide to Precision Cancer Management. Crit Rev Oncog 2023;28(2):45–62.

120. Sherley JL, Kelly TJ. Regulation of human thymidine kinase during the cell cycle. J Biol Chem 1988;263(17):8350–8.

121. Woodhouse DL. The composition of nucleic acids; the guanine and thymine content of nucleic acids isolated from normal tissues and animal tumours. Br J Cancer 1949;3(4):510–9.

122. Rasey JS, Grierson JR, Wiens LW, et al. Validation of FLT uptake as a measure of thymidine kinase-1 activity in A549 carcinoma cells. J Nucl Med 2002;43(9):1210–7.

123. Shields AF, Grierson JR, Dohmen BM, et al. Imaging proliferation in vivo with [F-18]FLT and positron emission tomography. Nat Med 1998;4(11):1334–6.

124. Chalkidou A, Landau DB, Odell EW, et al. Correlation between Ki-67 immunohistochemistry and 18F-fluorothymidine uptake in patients with cancer: A systematic review and meta-analysis. Eur J Cancer 2012;48(18):3499–513.

125. Garg G, Benchekroun MT, Abraham T. FDG-PET/CT in the Postoperative Period: Utility, Expected Findings, Complications, and Pitfalls. Semin Nucl Med 2017;47(6):579–94.

126. Varoquaux A, Rager O, Dulguerov P, et al. Diffusion-weighted and PET/MR Imaging after Radiation Therapy for Malignant Head and Neck Tumors. Radiographics 2015;35(5):1502–27.

127. Nappi AG, Santo G, Jonghi-Lavarini L, et al. Emerging Role of [(18)F]FLT PET/CT in Lymphoid Malignancies: A Review of Clinical Results. Hematol Rep 2024; 16(1):32–41.
128. Troost EG, Bussink J, Hoffmann AL, et al. 18F-FLT PET/CT for early response monitoring and dose escalation in oropharyngeal tumors. J Nucl Med 2010; 51(6):866–74.
129. Kishino T, Hoshikawa H, Nishiyama Y, et al. Usefulness of 3'-deoxy-3'-18F-fluorothymidine PET for predicting early response to chemoradiotherapy in head and neck cancer. J Nucl Med 2012;53(10):1521–7.
130. Hoeben BA, Troost EG, Span PN, et al. 18F-FLT PET during radiotherapy or chemoradiotherapy in head and neck squamous cell carcinoma is an early predictor of outcome. J Nucl Med 2013;54(4):532–40.
131. Emami Nejad A, Najafgholian S, Rostami A, et al. The role of hypoxia in the tumor microenvironment and development of cancer stem cell: a novel approach to developing treatment. Cancer Cell Int 2021;21(1):62.
132. Shi R, Liao C, Zhang Q. Hypoxia-driven effects in cancer: characterization, mechanisms, and therapeutic implications. Cells 2021;10(3).
133. Otrock ZK, Hatoum HA, Awada AH, et al. Hypoxia-inducible factor in cancer angiogenesis: structure, regulation and clinical perspectives. Crit Rev Oncol Hematol 2009;70(2):93–102.
134. Fu Z, Mowday AM, Smaill JB, et al. Tumour hypoxia-mediated immunosuppression: mechanisms and therapeutic approaches to improve cancer immunotherapy. Cells 2021;10(5).
135. Hasmim M, Noman MZ, Messai Y, et al. Cutting edge: Hypoxia-induced Nanog favors the intratumoral infiltration of regulatory T cells and macrophages via direct regulation of TGF-β1. J Immunol 2013;191(12):5802–6.
136. Westendorf AM, Skibbe K, Adamczyk A, et al. Hypoxia Enhances Immunosuppression by Inhibiting CD4+ Effector T Cell Function and Promoting Treg Activity. Cell Physiol Biochem 2017;41(4):1271–84.
137. Bhandari V, Hoey C, Liu LY, et al. Molecular landmarks of tumor hypoxia across cancer types. Nat Genet 2019;51(2):308–18.
138. Wang H, Jiang H, Van De Gucht M, et al. Hypoxic Radioresistance: Can ROS Be the Key to Overcome It? Cancers 2019;11(1).
139. Sachs RK, Chen PL, Hahnfeldt PJ, et al. DNA damage caused by ionizing radiation. Math Biosci 1992;112(2):271–303.
140. Rajendran JG, Schwartz DL, O'Sullivan J, et al. Tumor hypoxia imaging with [F-18] fluoromisonidazole positron emission tomography in head and neck cancer. Clin Cancer Res 2006;12(18):5435–41.
141. Jacobson O, Chen X. Interrogating tumor metabolism and tumor microenvironments using molecular positron emission tomography imaging. Theranostic approaches to improve therapeutics. Pharmacol Rev 2013;65(4):1214–56.
142. Noman MZ, Hasmim M, Messai Y, et al. Hypoxia: a key player in antitumor immune response. A Review in the Theme: Cellular Responses to Hypoxia. Am J Physiol Cell Physiol 2015;309(9):C569–79.
143. Rühle A, Grosu AL, Wiedenmann N, et al. Hypoxia dynamics on FMISO-PET in combination with PD-1/PD-L1 expression has an impact on the clinical outcome of patients with Head-and-neck Squamous Cell Carcinoma undergoing Chemoradiation. Theranostics 2020;10(20):9395–406.
144. Bandurska-Luque A, Löck S, Haase R, et al. FMISO-PET-based lymph node hypoxia adds to the prognostic value of tumor only hypoxia in HNSCC patients. Radiother Oncol 2019;130:97–103.

145. Löck S, Linge A, Seidlitz A, et al. Repeat FMISO-PET imaging weakly correlates with hypoxia-associated gene expressions for locally advanced HNSCC treated by primary radiochemotherapy. Radiother Oncol 2019;135:43–50.

146. Gouel P, Decazes P, Vera P, et al. Advances in PET and MRI imaging of tumor hypoxia. Front Med 2023;10:1055062.

147. Verel I, Visser GW, Boellaard R, et al. 89Zr immuno-PET: comprehensive procedures for the production of 89Zr-labeled monoclonal antibodies. J Nucl Med 2003;44(8):1271–81.

148. Meijs WE, Herscheid JD, Haisma HJ, et al. Evaluation of desferal as a bifunctional chelating agent for labeling antibodies with Zr-89. Int J Rad Appl Instrum A 1992;43(12):1443–7.

149. Meijs WE, Haisma HJ, Klok RP, et al. Zirconium-labeled monoclonal antibodies and their distribution in tumor-bearing nude mice. J Nucl Med 1997;38(1):112–8.

150. Jauw YW, Menke-van der Houven van Oordt CW, Hoekstra OS, et al. Immuno-positron emission tomography with zirconium-89-labeled monoclonal antibodies in oncology: what can we learn from initial clinical trials? Front Pharmacol 2016; 7:131.

151. Sarcan ET, Silindir-Gunay M, Ozer AY, et al. 89Zr as a promising radionuclide and it's applications for effective cancer imaging. J Radioanal Nucl Chem 2021;330(1):15–28.

152. Lee YJ, van den Berg NS, Duan H, et al. 89Zr-panitumumab Combined With 18F-FDG PET Improves Detection and Staging of Head and Neck Squamous Cell Carcinoma. Clin Cancer Res 2022;28(20):4425–34.

153. Börjesson PK, Jauw YW, Boellaard R, et al. Performance of immuno-positron emission tomography with zirconium-89-labeled chimeric monoclonal antibody U36 in the detection of lymph node metastases in head and neck cancer patients. Clin Cancer Res 2006;12(7 Pt 1):2133–40.

154. Eldeeb H, Macmillan C, Elwell C, et al. The effect of the surgical margins on the outcome of patients with head and neck squamous cell carcinoma: single institution experience. Cancer Biol Med 2012;9(1):29–33.

155. van Keulen S, Nishio N, Fakurnejad S, et al. The clinical application of fluorescence-guided surgery in head and neck cancer. J Nucl Med 2019; 60(6):758–63.

156. Lee Y-J, Krishnan G, Nishio N, et al. Intraoperative fluorescence-guided surgery in head and neck squamous cell carcinoma. Laryngoscope 2021;131(3): 529–34.

157. Rosenthal EL, Warram JM, de Boer E, et al. Successful translation of fluorescence navigation during oncologic surgery: a consensus report. J Nucl Med 2016;57(1):144–50.

158. de Kleijn BJ, Heldens GTN, Herruer JM, et al. Intraoperative imaging techniques to improve surgical resection margins of oropharyngeal squamous cell cancer: a comprehensive review of current literature. Cancers 2023;15(3).

159. Orosco RK, Tapia VJ, Califano JA, et al. Positive surgical margins in the 10 most common solid cancers. Sci Rep 2018;8(1):5686.

160. Gao RW, Teraphongphom NT, van den Berg NS, et al. Determination of tumor margins with surgical specimen mapping using near-infrared fluorescence. Cancer Res 2018;78(17):5144–54.

161. Krishnan G, van den Berg NS, Nishio N, et al. Fluorescent molecular imaging can improve intraoperative sentinel margin detection in oral squamous cell carcinoma. J Nucl Med 2022;63(8):1162–8.

162. Nishio N, van den Berg NS, van Keulen S, et al. Optical molecular imaging can differentiate metastatic from benign lymph nodes in head and neck cancer. Nat Commun 2019;10(1):5044.

163. Krishnan G, van den Berg NS, Nishio N, et al. Metastatic and sentinel lymph node mapping using intravenously delivered Panitumumab-IRDye800CW. Theranostics 2021;11(15):7188–98.

164. de Wit JG, Vonk J, Voskuil FJ, et al. EGFR-targeted fluorescence molecular imaging for intraoperative margin assessment in oral cancer patients: a phase II trial. Nat Commun 2023;14(1):4952.

165. Vonk J, de Wit JG, Voskuil FJ, et al. Epidermal growth factor receptor-targeted fluorescence molecular imaging for postoperative lymph node assessment in patients with oral cancer. J Nucl Med 2022;63(5):672–8.

166. Bou-Samra P, Muhammad N, Chang A, et al. Intraoperative molecular imaging: 3rd biennial clinical trials update. J Biomed Opt 2023;28(5):050901.

167. Wright GL, Haley C, Beckett ML, et al. Expression of prostate-specific membrane antigen in normal, benign, and malignant prostate tissues. Urol Oncol 1995;1(1):18–28.

168. Chang SS, Reuter VE, Heston WDW, et al. Five Different Anti-Prostate-specific Membrane Antigen (PSMA) Antibodies Confirm PSMA Expression in Tumor-associated Neovasculature1. Cancer Res 1999;59(13):3192–8.

169. Silver DA, Pellicer I, Fair WR, et al. Prostate-specific membrane antigen expression in normal and malignant human tissues. Clin Cancer Res 1997;3(1):81–5.

170. Klein Nulent TJW, van Es RJJ, Krijger GC, et al. Prostate-specific membrane antigen PET imaging and immunohistochemistry in adenoid cystic carcinoma-a preliminary analysis. Eur J Nucl Med Mol Imag 2017;44(10):1614–21.

171. Klein Nulent TJW, Valstar MH, Smit LA, et al. Prostate-specific membrane antigen (PSMA) expression in adenoid cystic carcinoma of the head and neck. BMC Cancer 2020;20(1):519.

172. de Keizer B, Krijger GC, Ververs FT, et al. 68Ga-PSMA PET-CT Imaging of Metastatic Adenoid Cystic Carcinoma. Nuclear Medicine and Molecular Imaging 2017;51(4):360–1.

173. Civan C, Kasper S, Berliner C, et al. PSMA-Directed Imaging and Therapy of Salivary Gland Tumors: A Single-Center Retrospective Study. J Nucl Med 2023;64(3):372–8.

174. Tan BF, Tan WCC, Wang FQ, et al. PSMA PET Imaging and Therapy in Adenoid Cystic Carcinoma and Other Salivary Gland Cancers: A Systematic Review. Cancers 2022;14(15).

175. Shamim SA, Kumar N, Arora G, et al. Comparison of 68Ga-PSMA-HBED-CC and 18F-FDG PET/CT in the Evaluation of Adenoid Cystic Carcinoma-A Prospective Study. Clin Nucl Med 2023;48(11):e509–15.

176. Terhaard CH, Lubsen H, Van der Tweel I, et al. Salivary gland carcinoma: independent prognostic factors for locoregional control, distant metastases, and overall survival: results of the Dutch head and neck oncology cooperative group. Head Neck 2004;26(8):681–92 [discussion 692-3].

177. Spiro RH. Distant metastasis in adenoid cystic carcinoma of salivary origin. Am J Surg 1997;174(5):495–8.

178. Sakthivel P, Thakar A, Prashanth A, et al. Prostate-specific membrane antigen expression in primary juvenile nasal angiofibroma-a pilot study. Clin Nucl Med 2020;45(3):195–9.

179. Sakthivel P, Thakar A, Arunraj ST, et al. Fusion 68Ga-Prostate-Specific Membrane Antigen PET/MRI on Postoperative Surveillance of Juvenile Nasal Angiofibroma. Clin Nucl Med 2020;45(7):e325–6.

180. Thakar A, Sakthivel P, Prashanth A, et al. Comparison of 68Ga-PSMA PET/CT and Contrast-Enhanced MRI on Residual Disease Assessment of Juvenile Nasal Angiofibroma. Clin Nucl Med 2020;45(4):308–9.

181. Sakthivel P, Thakar A, Prashanth A, et al. Clinical applications of (68)Ga-PSMA PET/CT on Residual Disease Assessment of Juvenile Nasopharyngeal Angiofibroma (JNA). Nucl Med Mol Imag 2020;54(1):63–4.

182. Mamelle G, Pampurik J, Luboinski B, et al. Lymph node prognostic factors in head and neck squamous cell carcinomas. Am J Surg 1994;168(5):494–8.

183. Singh P, Kaul P, Singhal T, et al. Role of sentinel lymph node drainage mapping for localization of contralateral lymph node metastasis in locally advanced oral squamous cell carcinoma - a prospective pilot study. Indian J Nucl Med Apr-Jun 2023;38(2):125–33.

184. Suresh GM, Koppad R, Prakash BV, et al. Prognostic indicators of oral squamous cell carcinoma. Ann Maxillofac Surg Jul-Dec 2019;9(2):364–70.

185. de Bree R, de Keizer B, Civantos FJ, et al. What is the role of sentinel lymph node biopsy in the management of oral cancer in 2020? Eur Arch Oto-Rhino-Laryngol 2021;278(9):3181–91.

186. de Bree R, Takes RP, Castelijns JA, et al. Advances in diagnostic modalities to detect occult lymph node metastases in head and neck squamous cell carcinoma. Head Neck 2015;37(12):1829–39.

187. Rudningen K, Sable KA, Glazer TA, et al. Contrast tomography (CT) performed to detect nodal metastasis for high-risk cutaneous squamous cell carcinomas of the head and neck has a high negative predictive value but a poor positive predictive value. JAAD Int 2023;13:37–8.

188. Skanjeti A, Dhomps A, Paschetta C, et al. Lymphoscintigraphy for sentinel node mapping in head and neck cancer. Semin Nucl Med 2021;51(1):39–49.

189. Schilling C, Stoeckli SJ, Haerle SK, et al. Sentinel European Node Trial (SENT): 3-year results of sentinel node biopsy in oral cancer. Eur J Cancer 2015;51(18):2777–84.

190. Kokoska MS, Olson G, Kelemen PR, et al. The use of lymphoscintigraphy and pet in the management of head and neck melanoma. Otolaryngology-Head Neck Surg (Tokyo) 2001;125(3):213–20.

191. Pfeiffer ML, Ozgur OK, Myers JN, et al. Sentinel lymph node biopsy for ocular adnexal melanoma. Acta Ophthalmol 2017;95(4):e323–8.

192. Alkureishi LW, Burak Z, Alvarez JA, et al. Joint practice guidelines for radionuclide lymphoscintigraphy for sentinel node localization in oral/oropharyngeal squamous cell carcinoma. Ann Surg Oncol 2009;16(11):3190–210.

193. Mahieu R, de Maar JS, Nieuwenhuis ER, et al. New developments in imaging for sentinel lymph node biopsy in early-stage oral cavity squamous cell carcinoma. Cancers 2020;12(10).

194. Munn LL, Padera TP. Imaging the lymphatic system. Microvasc Res 2014;96:55–63.

195. Azem O, King K, Joshi NP, et al. Evaluation of sentinel lymph node drainage patterns in early-stage oral cavity cancer. Int J Radiat Oncol Biol Phys 2023;117(2, Supplement):e564.

196. Liu M, Wang SJ, Yang X, et al. Diagnostic efficacy of sentinel lymph node biopsy in early oral squamous cell carcinoma: a meta-analysis of 66 studies. PLoS One 2017;12(1):e0170322.

197. Garau LM, Di Gregorio F, Nonne G, et al. Measures of performance for sentinel lymph node biopsy in oro-oropharyngeal squamous cell carcinoma: a systematic review and meta-analysis. Clin Transl Imag 2023;11(6):599–614.
198. de Veij Mestdagh PD, Walraven I, Vogel WV, et al. SPECT/CT-guided elective nodal irradiation for head and neck cancer is oncologically safe and less toxic: A potentially practice-changing approach. Radiother Oncol 2020;147:56–63.
199. Reinders FCJ, de Ridder M, Doornaert PAH, Raaijmakers C, Philippens MEP. Individual elective lymph node irradiation for the reduction of complications in head and neck cancer patients (iNode): A phase-I feasibility trial protocol. Clin Translat Rad Oncol 2023;39:100574.
200. de Veij Mestdagh PD, Schreuder WH, Vogel WV, et al. Mapping of sentinel lymph node drainage using SPECT/CT to tailor elective nodal irradiation in head and neck cancer patients (SUSPECT-2): a single-center prospective trial. BMC Cancer 2019;19(1):1110.
201. Almeida JRd, Parulekar WR, Christopoulos A, et al. CCTG HN11: SPECT-CT guided elective contralateral neck treatment (SELECT) for patients with lateralized oropharyngeal cancer—A phase III randomized controlled trial. J Clin Oncol 2023;41(16_suppl):TPS6114.
202. Swetter SM, Tsao H, Bichakjian CK, et al. Guidelines of care for the management of primary cutaneous melanoma. J Am Acad Dermatol 2019;80(1):208–50.
203. Cramer JD, Sridharan S, Ferris RL, et al. Sentinel lymph node biopsy versus elective neck dissection for stage I to II oral cavity cancer. Laryngoscope 2019;129(1):162–9.
204. Krag D, Weaver D, Ashikaga T, et al. The sentinel node in breast cancer–a multicenter validation study. N Engl J Med 1998;339(14):941–6.
205. Jimenez-Heffernan A, Ellmann A, Sado H, et al. Results of a prospective multicenter international atomic energy agency sentinel node trial on the value of SPECT/CT over planar imaging in various malignancies. J Nucl Med 2015;56(9):1338–44.
206. Remenschneider AK, Dilger AE, Wang Y, et al. The predictive value of single-photon emission computed tomography/computed tomography for sentinel lymph node localization in head and neck cutaneous malignancy. Laryngoscope 2015;125(4):877–82.
207. Health NIo. Comparing Sentinel Lymph Node (SLN) Biopsy with standard neck dissection for patients with early-stage oral cavity cancer. Available at: https://clinicaltrials.gov/study/NCT04333537. [Accessed 30 January 2024].
208. Cheng Z, Ma J, Yin L, et al. Non-invasive molecular imaging for precision diagnosis of metastatic lymph nodes: opportunities from preclinical to clinical applications. Eur J Nucl Med Mol Imag 2023;50(4):1111–33.
209. Li S, Cheng D, He L, et al. Recent progresses in NIR-I/II fluorescence imaging for surgical navigation. Front Bioeng Biotechnol 2021;9:768698.
210. Li H, Kim D, Yao Q, et al. Activity-Based NIR enzyme fluorescent probes for the diagnosis of tumors and image-guided surgery. Angew Chem Int Ed Engl 2021;60(32):17268–89.
211. Kennedy GT, Azari FS, Bernstein E, et al. Targeted intraoperative molecular imaging for localizing nonpalpable tumors and quantifying resection margin distances. JAMA Surg 2021;156(11):1043–50.
212. Lamberts LE, Koch M, de Jong JS, et al. Tumor-specific uptake of fluorescent bevacizumab–IRDye800CW microdosing in patients with primary breast cancer: a phase I feasibility study. Clin Cancer Res 2017;23(11):2730–41.

213. "Panitumumab-IRDye800 and 89Zr-panitumumab in identifying metastatic lymph nodes in patients with squamous cell head and neck cancer.". ClinicalTrials.gov identifier: NCT03733210. Available at: https://www.clinicaltrials.gov/study/NCT03733210?cond=Head%2520and%2520Neck&term=Lymph%2520Node%2520Metastasis&intr=imaging&rank=9. [Accessed 11 January 2024].

214. Hermans R. Head and neck cancer: how imaging predicts treatment outcome. Cancer Imag 2006;6(Spec No A):S145–53.

215. Awan KH, Patil S. Efficacy of autofluorescence imaging as an adjunctive technique for examination and detection of oral potentially malignant disorders: a systematic review. J Contemp Dent Pract 2015;16(9):744–9.

216. Ni XG, Wang GQ, Zhang QQ. Narrow band imaging versus autofluorescence imaging for head and neck squamous cell carcinoma detection: a prospective study. J Laryngol Otol 2016;130(11):1001–6.

217. Subramanian V, Ragunath K. Advanced endoscopic imaging: a review of commercially available technologies. Clin Gastroenterol Hepatol 2014;12(3): 368–76.e1.

218. Hughes OR, Stone N, Kraft M, et al. Optical and molecular techniques to identify tumor margins within the larynx. Head Neck 2010;32(11):1544–53.

219. Piazza C, Dessouky O, Peretti G, et al. Narrow-band imaging: a new tool for evaluation of head and neck squamous cell carcinomas. Review of the literature. Acta Otorhinolaryngol Ital 2008;28(2):49–54.

220. Cosway B, Drinnan M, Paleri V. Narrow band imaging for the diagnosis of head and neck squamous cell carcinoma: A systematic review. Head Neck 2016; 38(S1):E2358–67.

221. Chu P-Y, Tsai T-L, Tai S-K, et al. Effectiveness of narrow band imaging in patients with oral squamous cell carcinoma after treatment. Head Neck 2012;34(2): 155–61.

222. Watanabe A, Tsujie H, Taniguchi M, et al. Laryngoscopic detection of pharyngeal carcinoma in situ with narrowband imaging. Laryngoscope 2006;116(4): 650–4.

223. Katada C, Nakayama M, Tanabe S, et al. Narrow band imaging for detecting metachronous superficial oropharyngeal and hypopharyngeal squamous cell carcinomas after chemoradiotherapy for head and neck cancers. Laryngoscope 2008;118(10):1787–90.

224. Dippold S, Becker C, Nusseck M, et al. Narrow band imaging: a tool for endoscopic examination of patients with laryngeal papillomatosis. Ann Otol Rhinol Laryngol 2015;124(11):886–92.

225. Muto M, Nakane M, Katada C, et al. Squamous cell carcinoma in situ at oropharyngeal and hypopharyngeal mucosal sites. Cancer 2004;101(6):1375–81.

226. Ugumori T, Muto M, Hayashi R, et al. Prospective study of early detection of pharyngeal superficial carcinoma with the narrowband imaging laryngoscope. Head Neck 2009;31(2):189–94.

227. Katada C, Tanabe S, Koizumi W, et al. Narrow band imaging for detecting superficial squamous cell carcinoma of the head and neck in patients with esophageal squamous cell carcinoma. Endoscopy 2010;42(03):185–90.

228. Matsuba H, Katada C, Masaki T, et al. Diagnosis of the extent of advanced oropharyngeal and hypopharyngeal cancers by narrow band imaging with magnifying endoscopy. Laryngoscope 2011;121(4):753–9.

229. Piazza C, Cocco D, Del Bon F, et al. Narrow band imaging and high definition television in evaluation of oral and oropharyngeal squamous cell cancer: A prospective study. Oral Oncol 2010;46(4):307–10.

230. Syba J, Trnkova K, Dostalova L, et al. Comparison of narrow-band imaging with autofluorescence imaging for endoscopic detection of squamous cell carcinoma of the tonsil. Eur Arch Oto-Rhino-Laryngol 2023;280(11):5073–80.

231. Chabrillac E, Dupret-Bories A, Vairel B, et al. Narrow-band imaging in oncologic otorhinolaryngology: State of the art. Eur Ann Otorhinolaryngol Head Neck Dis 2021;138(6):451–8.

232. Vilaseca I, Valls-Mateus M, Nogués A, et al. Usefulness of office examination with narrow band imaging for the diagnosis of head and neck squamous cell carcinoma and follow-up of premalignant lesions. Head Neck 2017;39(9): 1854–63.

233. Valls-Mateus M, Nogués-Sabaté A, Blanch JL, et al. Narrow band imaging for head and neck malignancies: Lessons learned from mistakes. Head Neck 2018;40(6):1164–73.

234. Vonk J, de Wit JG, Voskuil FJ, et al. Improving oral cavity cancer diagnosis and treatment with fluorescence molecular imaging. Oral Dis 2021;27(1):21–6.

235. Marsden M, Weyers BW, Bec J, et al. Intraoperative margin assessment in oral and oropharyngeal cancer using label-free fluorescence lifetime imaging and machine learning. IEEE (Inst Electr Electron Eng) Trans Biomed Eng 2021; 68(3):857–68.

236. de Wit JG, van Schaik JE, Voskuil FJ, et al. Comparison of narrow band and fluorescence molecular imaging to improve intraoperative tumour margin assessment in oral cancer surgery. Oral Oncol 2022;134:106099.

237. Voskuil FJ, de Jongh SJ, Hooghiemstra WTR, et al. Fluorescence-guided imaging for resection margin evaluation in head and neck cancer patients using cetuximab-800CW: A quantitative dose-escalation study. Theranostics 2020; 10(9):3994–4005.

238. Weyers BW, Marsden M, Sun T, et al. Fluorescence lifetime imaging for intraoperative cancer delineation in transoral robotic surgery. Translational Biophotonics 2019;1(1–2). e201900017.

239. Jiang JX, Keating JJ, Jesus EM, et al. Optimization of the enhanced permeability and retention effect for near-infrared imaging of solid tumors with indocyanine green. Am J Nucl Med Mol Imaging 2015;5(4):390–400.

240. De Ravin E, Venkatesh S, Harmsen S, et al. Indocyanine green fluorescence-guided surgery in head and neck cancer: A systematic review. Am J Otolaryngol 2022;43(5):103570.

241. Namikawa T, Iwabu J, Munekage M, et al. Evolution of photodynamic medicine based on fluorescence image-guided diagnosis using indocyanine green and 5-aminolevulinic acid. Surg Today 2020;50(8):821–31.

242. Schupper AJ, Hadjipanayis C. Use of intraoperative fluorophores. Neurosurg Clin 2021/01/01/2021;32(1):55–64.

243. Lee JY, Thawani JP, Pierce J, et al. Intraoperative near-infrared optical imaging can localize gadolinium-enhancing gliomas during surgery. Neurosurgery 2016; 79(6):856–71.

244. Arens C, Reussner D, Woenkhaus J, et al. Indirect fluorescence laryngoscopy in the diagnosis of precancerous and cancerous laryngeal lesions. Eur Arch Oto-Rhino-Laryngol 2007;264(6):621–6.

245. Leunig A, Betz CS, Mehlmann M, et al. Detection of squamous cell carcinoma of the oral cavity by imaging 5-aminolevulinic acid-induced protoporphyrin IX fluorescence. Laryngoscope 2000;110(1):78–83.

246. Filip P, Lerner DK, Kominsky E, et al. 5-Aminolevulinic acid fluorescence-guided surgery in head and neck squamous cell carcinoma. Laryngoscope 2024. https://doi.org/10.1002/lary.30910.

247. Gillies RJ, Kinahan PE, Hricak H. Radiomics: images are more than pictures, they are data. Radiology 2016;278(2):563–77.

248. Shur JD, Doran SJ, Kumar S, et al. Radiomics in oncology: a practical guide. Radiographics 2021;41(6):1717–32.

249. Ling X, Alexander GS, Molitoris J, et al. Identification of CT-based non-invasive radiomic biomarkers for overall survival prediction in oral cavity squamous cell carcinoma. Sci Rep 2023;13(1):21774.

250. Corti A, De Cecco L, Cavalieri S, et al. MRI-based radiomic prognostic signature for locally advanced oral cavity squamous cell carcinoma: development, testing and comparison with genomic prognostic signatures. Biomark Res 2023; 11(1):69.

251. Jiang S, Locatello LG, Maggiore G, et al. Radiomics-based analysis in the prediction of occult lymph node metastases in patients with oral cancer: a systematic review. J Clin Med 2023;12(15).

252. Glogauer J, Kohanzadeh A, Feit A, et al. The use of radiomic features to predict human papillomavirus (hpv) status in head and neck tumors: a review. Cureus 2023;15(8):e44476.

253. Boot PA, Mes SW, de Bloeme CM, et al. Magnetic resonance imaging based radiomics prediction of Human Papillomavirus infection status and overall survival in oropharyngeal squamous cell carcinoma. Oral Oncol 2023;137:106307.

254. Bos P, van den Brekel MWM, Gouw ZAR, et al. Clinical variables and magnetic resonance imaging-based radiomics predict human papillomavirus status of oropharyngeal cancer. Head Neck 2021;43(2):485–95.

255. Giannitto C, Marvaso G, Botta F, et al. Association of quantitative MRI-based radiomic features with prognostic factors and recurrence rate in oropharyngeal squamous cell carcinoma. Neoplasma 2020;67(6):1437–46.

256. Marzi S, Piludu F, Avanzolini I, et al. Multifactorial model based on DWI-radiomics to determine HPV status in oropharyngeal squamous cell carcinoma. Appl Sci 2022;12(14):7244.

257. Park YM, Lim JY, Koh YW, et al. Machine learning and magnetic resonance imaging radiomics for predicting human papilloma virus status and prognostic factors in oropharyngeal squamous cell carcinoma. Head Neck 2022;44(4):897–903.

258. Altinok O, Guvenis A. Interpretable radiomics method for predicting human papillomavirus status in oropharyngeal cancer using Bayesian networks. Phys Med 2023;114:102671.

259. Kowalchuk RO, Van Abel KM, Yin LX, et al. Correlation between radiographic and pathologic lymph node involvement and extranodal extension via CT and PET in HPV-associated oropharyngeal cancer. Oral Oncol 2021;123:105625.

260. Lin CH, Yan JL, Yap WK, et al. Prognostic value of interim CT-based peritumoral and intratumoral radiomics in laryngeal and hypopharyngeal cancer patients undergoing definitive radiotherapy. Radiother Oncol 2023;189:109938.

261. Nguyen TM, Bertolus C, Giraud P, et al. A radiomics approach to identify immunologically active tumor in patients with head and neck squamous cell carcinomas. Cancers 2023;15(22).

262. Lu HJ, Shen CY, Chiu YW, et al. Radiomic biomarkers for platinum-refractory head and neck cancer in the era of immunotherapy. Oral Dis 2024.

263. Ren J, Yang G, Song Y, et al. Machine learning-based MRI radiomics for assessing the level of tumor infiltrating lymphocytes in oral tongue squamous cell carcinoma: a pilot study. BMC Med Imag 2024;24(1):33.

264. Almangush A, Leivo I, Mäkitie AA. Overall assessment of tumor-infiltrating lymphocytes in head and neck squamous cell carcinoma: time to take notice. Acta Otolaryngol 2020;140(3):246–8.

265. Mahmood H, Shaban M, Rajpoot N, et al. Artificial Intelligence-based methods in head and neck cancer diagnosis: an overview. Br J Cancer 2021;124(12): 1934–40.

266. Woo C, Jo KH, Sohn B, et al. Development and testing of a machine learning model using (18)F-Fluorodeoxyglucose PET/CT-derived metabolic parameters to classify human papillomavirus status in oropharyngeal squamous carcinoma. Korean J Radiol 2023;24(1):51–61.

267. Seidler M, Forghani B, Reinhold C, et al. Dual-Energy CT texture analysis with machine learning for the evaluation and characterization of cervical lymphadenopathy. Comput Struct Biotechnol J 2019;17:1009–15.

268. Klein S, Wuerdemann N, Demers I, et al. Predicting HPV association using deep learning and regular H&E stains allows granular stratification of oropharyngeal cancer patients. NPJ Digit Med 2023;6(1):152.

269. Bibault JE, Giraud P. Deep learning for automated segmentation in radiotherapy: a narrative review. Br J Radiol 2024;97(1153):13–20.

270. Chen H, Ma X, Rives H, et al. Trust in machine learning driven clinical decision support tools among otolaryngologists. Laryngoscope 2024. https://doi.org/10. 1002/lary.31260.

Trends and Future Directions in Margin Analysis for Head and Neck Cancers

Ramez Philips, MD[a,*], Pratyusha Yalamanchi, MD[a],
Michael C. Topf, MD, MSCI[a,b]

KEYWORDS

- Margin analysis • Frozen section • Molecular margins
- Intraoperative communication • Optical imaging • Artificial intelligence
- Optical coherence tomography • Fluorescence

KEY POINTS

- Negative margins are 25 mm away from the tumor periphery on histopathologic examination and oncologic significance varies by primary site; 1 to 2 mm narrow margins are accepted for early-stage glottic cancer.
- Frozen specimens margins are utilized.
  - These may be sampled from the tumor bed (defect-driven) or the tumor itself (specimen-based).
  - Specimen-driven approaches improve rates of local control particularly in oral cavity but are resource intensive.
  - Bony/adipose margins are unreliable on frozen pathology.
- Close margins differ by primary site and surgical modality (eg, transoral robotic surgery for human papillomavirus + oropharynx cancer) and less than 3 mm in combination with adverse features have been reported to predict worse oncologic outcomes.
- Significance of positive frozen margins
  - Reresection, when feasible to a negative margin, is performed but may be representative of aggressive tumor biology and merit adjuvant therapy.
  - Carcinoma in situ and severe dysplasia on frozen analysis are currently variably managed.

INTRODUCTION

The standard of care for the treatment head and neck squamous cell carcinomas (HNSCCs) is surgical resection followed by pathology-driven adjuvant treatment.

[a] Department of Otolaryngology–Head and Neck Surgery, Vanderbilt University Medical Center, 1211 Medical Center Drive, Nashville, TN 37232, USA; [b] Vanderbilt University School of Engineering, 1211 Medical Center Drive, Nashville, TN 37232, USA
* Corresponding author. 1211 Medical Center Drive, Nashville, TN 37232.
E-mail address: ramez.philip@vumc.org

Surgery provides en bloc resection of the tumor while preserving critical functions of the head and neck. The presence of invasive carcinoma at the periphery of a surgical specimen is associated with poor local control and decreased survival.[1,2] If unable to be reresected, positive margins require more aggressive adjuvant treatment with the addition of chemotherapy to radiation therapy.[3,4] To achieve negative margins, surgeons resect a margin of normal-appearing tissue around the tumor as vision and palpation alone cannot detect microscopic tumor cells. Following resection, assessment of margins is commonly performed using frozen section analysis (FSA). A timely diagnosis from the pathologist can lead to further reresection in the case of a positive or close margin, with the goal of negative intraoperative and final margins. In this review, the authors define negative margins, describe current practices, and highlight innovation in margin analysis.

CURRENT PRACTICES AND CHALLENGES IN MARGIN ANALYSIS
Defining a Negative Margin

While the primary goal of oncologic surgery is complete tumor resection with a circumferential margin of normal tissue, the threshold for a close or positive margin within head and neck oncology continues to be debated. The National Comprehensive Cancer Network (NCCN) guidelines define a negative margin as invasive carcinoma ≥5 mm away from the specimen periphery on histopathologic examination, while a "close" margin is less than 5 mm.[5] A positive margin is defined as the presence of carcinoma in situ (CIS) or invasive carcinoma at the edge of the inked tumor specimen. These data was largely based on early studies on oral cavity tumors indicating increased risk of recurrence with tumors within 0.5 mm of the surgical margin.[1,6] However, the optimal surgical margin distance remains a topic of debate.[7,8] A study by Singh and colleagues[7] including 451 tongue cancers found significant locoregional free survival benefit between 2.1 mm and 7.5 mm margins compared to less than 2.0 mm margins (hazard ratio [HR], 3.42; 95% confidence interval [CI], 1.65–7.09; $P = .001$). Based on these data, the authors argue that we should reconsider margin distance of less than 2 mm as involved and greater than 7.5 mm as adequate. A 2019 survey of American Head and Neck Society members found that only approximately half of surveyed surgeons used 5 mm or greater on microscopic evaluation as the specified radial margin distance that they considered a negative margin in oral cavity resections.[9] The remaining surgeons used a microscopic cutoff of 1 cm gross margin (22.8%) or 'other' cutoffs (~8%) defined as 1 to 3 mm microscopically or 1.5 cm grossly as the definition of a negative margin. Most surgeons (62%) considered CIS at the specimen periphery to be a positive margin, while 40.8% considered severe dysplasia. Despite recent studies demonstrating that CIS and severe dysplasia at the resection margin negatively impact survival,[9–11] NCCN guidelines do not explicitly recommend adjuvant therapy if only CIS is found at the specimen margin.[5]

While margin status definitions continue to be debated, the poor prognostic implications of positive margins are well established. Positive margins were defined as "less than 5 mm" in the European Organization for Research and Treatment of Cancer (# 22931) study and "at the surgical margin" in the Radiation Therapy Oncology Group 9501 study. Data from both phase III trials demonstrated that in patients with oral cavity, oropharynx, larynx, and hypopharynx malignancies, positive margin and/or extranodal extension patients treated with adjuvant chemoradiotherapy (compared to radiation alone) had significant improvement in overall survival and locoregional failure rates.[3,4,12]

Of note, the earlier explanation of margin status assumes a binary definition and does not consider cellular changes on the spectrum from normal to malignant tissue.

Margin status in head and neck cancer is complicated by tumor and stroma biology. To better classify this spectral landscape, the worst pattern of invasion (WPOI) classification was developed to characterize tumor aggression at the surgical margins.[13,14] The WPOI classification describes the tumor front from broad pushing to invasive islands, and tumor satellites. Higher classifications of WPOI act as a surrogate for aggressive tumor biology and have been associated with worse local recurrence and overall and disease-free survival.[15–17] The integration of WPOI with margin distance highlights the intersection of tumor biology and optimal surgical tumor extirpation. Prior treatment can also lead to difficulty in understanding margins; for example, induction/neoadjuvant treatment before surgical resection or recurrent disease after prior treatment may complicate the assessment of the surgical margin.

Frozen Section Analysis

Intraoperative FSA is considered the standard of care for rapid intraoperative assessment of resection margins. Virtually all head and neck surgeons (99%) report using FSA regularly with the goal of maximizing complete tumor removal in a single operative setting and minimizing the likelihood of a final positive surgical margin and need for additional surgery and/or adjuvant therapy.[18]

After tumor extirpation, the specimen is transported to the pathology laboratory for FSA to ensure adequate removal of the cancer with clear surgical margins. First, a resected tumor specimen is anatomically oriented and grossly inspected by the pathologist. Margins that are close on gross examination of the specimen are then sectioned for FSA. Fresh tissue is frozen in a cryostat machine, thinly sliced, attached to a glass slide, and stained for histopathologic analysis. Multiple studies confirm the accuracy and utility of intraoperative FSA in head and neck cancer surgery.[19–25]

Tumor Bed Versus Specimen-Driven Approach

FSA is performed via (1) a specimen-based approach in which tissue is analyzed directly from the resection specimen or (2) a tumor bed approach, in which samples are taken from the tumor bed at the surgeon's discretion. While there is increasing evidence to support improved oncologic outcomes with the specimen-based approach, 45% of surveyed head and neck surgeons utilize tumor bed margins for oral cavity oncologic resections with many citing feasibility in daily practice.[9] When obtaining a margin from the tumor bed, surgeons often obtain circumferential margins based on anatomic subsites surrounding the tumor. The anatomic location of these margins is communicated to the pathologist. After histopathologic assessment of the specimen, the results are communicated back to the surgeon. Tumor bed margins offer timely information but have been increasingly critiqued due to sampling bias, localization challenges, and providing insufficient information regarding distance of the tumor to the resection margin.

In a specimen-based FSA margins protocol, the specimen is taken down to the pathology laboratory where it is oriented. Gross examination and palpation can indicate areas at highest risk of positive or close margins. Intraoperative tissue cuts or tears that are not true margins can also be communicated in this handoff. After inking the specimen margin, the pathologist can 'bread loaf' the specimen to obtain frozen sections based on areas of highest risk. The margins are taken off the main resection specimen. These sections can identify both tumor margin status and distance. Any positive margins can be communicated with the surgeon to allow for reresection.

Thorough histologic evaluation, with slides performed at multiple levels of the margins at the time of frozen sections, has been demonstrated to have a reduction in the false-negative rate for intraoperative margin assessment.[26] Most importantly, a specimen-based approach to margin analysis has been shown to improve oncologic outcomes.[27] The authors attribute worse local control in tumor bed margins to narrower margin clearance and lower sensitivity of identifying positive glossectomy margins. A clinical trial by Amit and colleagues[28] provided evidence for the low sensitivity of identifying positive glossectomy margins when relying on margins from the tumor bed. In an analysis of 71 patients with HNSCC receiving surgery, wide negative margin rate was 84% compared to 55% (P=.02) in patients undergoing specimen-based versus tumor-based margin analysis. The primary limitation of the specimen-based FSA approach is the time and labor-intensive nature of the approach as this often requires the surgeon to travel to a variably located surgical pathology laboratory to handoff the specimen. To this point, FSA has also been suggested to be cost-intensive with unclear benefits.[29,30] The investigators have found that assessing margin status using FSA has a cost-benefit ratio of 12:1 and impacts rate of free margins or adjuvant treatment only 2.3% and 0.7% of the time, respectively.[29]

Though intraoperative FSA is regularly used in head and neck oncologic surgery, the oncologic benefit of revising positive margins remains less clear. A study by Nentwig and colleagues[31] reported that 42.1% of frozen section positive margins remain positive despite immediate reresection. FSA-guided resections revised from positive to clear margins based on reresection remain at greater risk of local failure than initially cleared margins.[32-34] When compared to resected tumors with final positive margins, tumors with initial positive margins revised to negative did not show a significant association with improved locoregional survival (R1 vs R1 to R0; HR = 1.523; 95% CI,0.992–2.338, P = . 055), questioning the effect of FSA on local recurrence.[35] The aforementioned studies likely reflect inherent tumor biology that is not evident on gross examination, and merit consideration of adjuvant therapy even when margins have been cleared with FSA-guided reresection. Despite the risk of local failure, the effect of positive initial margins, with subsequent negative final margins, on overall survival continues to be a subject of debate.[36,37] Ultimately, final negative margins remain of utmost importance for prognosis.[38] Further investigations regarding the oncologic benefit of reresection under FSA guidance is indicated as we continue to clarify definitions of adequate margins and reporting standards and FSA techniques.

Primary Site–Specific Margin Analysis

Bony margins

The prognostic value of margins in head and neck cancer is also dependent upon primary tumor site, mode of resection, and ease of histopathologic analysis. For instance, the extent of osseous resection in composite oral cavity resections is determined by surgeons upon review of preoperative imaging and gross intraoperative examination. The high mineral content is not traditionally amenable to FSA and requires decalcification for histologic assessment. However, cytologic assessment of bone marrow scrapings and sampling of cancellous (as opposed to cortical) bone from the tumor bed has been reported.[26]

Larynx

While a negative margin for oral cavity carcinoma is most frequently reported as ≥5 mm away from the tumor periphery on histopathologic examination, there is consensus that appropriate glottic resection margins, often obtained by transoral laser surgery, may be as limited as 1 to 2 mm with no impact on locoregional recurrence.[39] This has been attributed to the overall excellent prognosis of early-stage glottic cancer, as well as possible specimen shrinkage. Defect-driven approaches to intraoperative glottic margin surveillance are typically utilized with an emphasis on tissue preservation to optimize voice outcomes. In contrast, surgical positive margins for higher stage glottic cancers particularly those involving the anterior commissure have repeatedly been shown to be associated with decreased local control rates.[40–43]

Human papillomavirus + oropharynx

With the increased incidence of human papillomavirus (HPV)–related disease and the advent of transoral robotic surgery, margin assessment in oropharyngeal disease has garnered significant attention.[44] Special attention must be paid to deep margins, rather than mucosal margins, as they are more likely to be close and challenging to assess and resect.[2,32] The superior constrictor and adjacent parapharyngeal fat act as a natural barrier for the spread of the disease at the deep margin. Anatomic studies have revealed the thickness of the lateral oropharyngeal wall to be often less than 5 mm.[45,46] Therefore, the ability to obtain a 5-mm deep margin in lateral oropharyngeal tumors may not be possible.[44,45] Beyond anatomic considerations, HPV-related tumors have improved oncologic outcomes compared to HPV-unrelated tumors and are perhaps more likely to be forgiving with margin distance.[47,48] Iyer and colleagues[49] identified no difference in 5-year overall survival in patients with close/positive versus negative margins in HPV-related tumors, whereas HPV-negative tumors with close/positive margins had significantly worse overall survival. Disparate institution practice patterns, varied resection techniques, and nonuniformity in reporting of margin status make multi-institution comparisons of the oncologic outcomes associated with different head and neck primary sites challenging and merit future investigation.

Margin Relocation

If a close or positive margin is identified intraoperatively on FSA, the surgeon relies on verbal communication provided during a phone call with the pathologist to relocate the margin and resect additional tissue. Successful reresection requires the surgeon to (1) identify the exact location on the specimen where the positive margin was sampled and (2) locate the anatomic point in the resection bed that corresponds to the location of the positive margin. The surgeon must do so without any visual aid, which is difficult due to the complex 3-dimensional (3D) anatomy in the head and neck. Reported mean relocation error of a margin is 10.3 to 20.6 mm.[50,51] Surprisingly, only 20% of reresections contain further malignancy.[52] Challenges with margin relocation is one reason why reresection does not improve patient outcomes.[32,33,53,54] Both surgeons and pathologists recognize the importance of leveraging new technology to improve margin relocation.[55]

INNOVATION IN MARGIN ANALYSIS
Enhancing Intraoperative Communication

One of the main challenges in specimen-based margin assessment is accurate communication between the surgeon and the pathologist regarding the anatomic location and type (perpendicular/radial vs shave/en face) of obtained margins to enhance relocation.[51,56] Novel 3D scanning technology and computer-aided design (CAD) software provides improved intraoperative communication between the surgeon and the pathologist.[57,58] After tumor resection, the ex vivo specimen is scanned using a 3D-structured light scanner to reconstruct the surface topography of the specimen. This image is then processed and exported into CAD software. Simultaneously, the specimen is handed off to the pathology team where it is inked, sectioned, and frozen in preparation for specimen-based margin analysis. The inked areas on the specimen can then be translated on the 3D model using a digital airbrush (**Fig. 1**). After results of specimen-based margins are obtained, communication between the

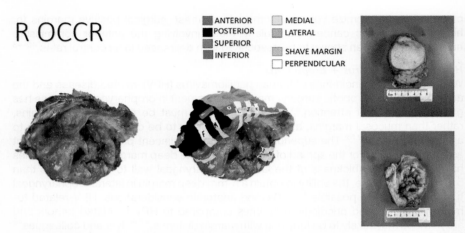

Fig. 1. Screen image of a virtual 3-dimensional specimen map (*left*) of a right oral cavity composite resection with airbrushed colors depicting orientation and margin type. Obtained margins are labeled with letters. Gross photographs are depicted on the right.

surgeon and the pathologist can be facilitated using the 3D specimen map displayed on the overhead operating room monitors via remote videoconferencing without the surgeon physically traveling to the gross pathology laboratory. Preliminary studies have demonstrated feasibility of incorporating this technology into the margin assessment workflow.[57,58]

This protocol can be further enhanced by augmented reality (AR). AR can be used to align a hologram of the 3D specimen map to patient's tumor bed defect.[59] In a prior cadaver study, surgeons were able to align the 3D specimen hologram with a mean relocation error of 4 mm (range 1–15 mm) (**Fig. 2**). Though this technology provides promise in the avenue of intraoperative communication to improve margin reliability, it is not without limitations. Primarily, there exists a learning curve, which can translate

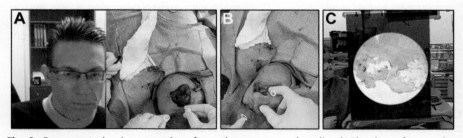

Fig. 2. Representative images taken from the augmented reality (AR) teleconference between the surgeon and the pathologist for the resection of basosquamous carcinoma of the upper lip. The field of view reflects what the surgeon sees through the HoloLens headset. (*A*) In the right panel, the upper lip and partial rhinectomy 3-dimensional (3D) specimen is oriented by the surgeon into the resection bed. Margin sampling sites for frozen section analysis are denoted by virtual annotation in blue ink. In the left panel, the pathologist observes the same surgical field and AR elements as the surgeon and engages in a 2-way verbal communication. (*B*) The right nasal skin margin sampling site is identified by the surgeon and correlated to the annotated virtual 3D specimen. (*C*) A 2-dimensional image of the right nasal skin margin hematoxylin and eosin (H&E) slide is presented by the surgeon. The pathologist interprets the slide and reports a negative margin on frozen section analysis.

into increased length of time (7–8 minutes) to reporting margin results.[57,58] An important limitation is the effect of tissue shrinkage on realignment of the tumor using AR technology. Tissue shrinkage can alter tumor shape, rendering accurate realignment of specimen difficult.[60–62] Further studies are required to incorporate 3D modeling and AR into the standard workflow.

Molecular Margins

As it stands, current margin analysis is based on distance of invasive tumor cells from specimen edge on histopathology. Recently, there has been major development in our understanding of the molecular landscape of HNSCC and adjacent "normal" tissue. Incorporating molecular margins could provide a more accurate assessment of tumor biology at the specimen periphery. Currently, research in molecular margins has been based on varying methods of assessing genetic/epigenetic mutations to downstream changes in protein expression.[63] Early mutations in head and neck cancer may not manifest histologically and thus go undetected. This contributes to the increased risk of local failure in the setting of negative histopathologic margins. Identifying early mutations in oncogenesis at the tumor periphery may provide improved understanding of tumor extent. An important known early mutation in tumorigenesis occurs in TP53. TP53 gene codes for p53, a tumor suppressing transcriptional factor, labeled the 'guardian of the genome' due its important function in maintaining the cell cycle.[64] TP53 is mutated in up to 78% of HNSCCs and occurs early and is pivotal in molecular tumorigenesis.[65] Studies utilizing polymerase chain reaction (PCR)–based technology have identified TP53 mutations at a histologically clear specimen margin to be important predictor of locoregional recurrence.[66,67] When controlling for other clinicopathologic factors, a positive molecular at a negative histologic margin remains independently associated with locoregional recurrence. Despite the positive results using PCR technology, protein-based analysis using immunohistochemistry (IHC) has not shown significant correlation between positive molecular margins and oncological outcomes.[68,69]

Other molecular markers such as cyclin D1, a G1 checkpoint–regulating oncogene, and eukaryotic translocation initiation factor 4E (eIF4E), a factor involved in protein synthesis, have been investigated as molecular markers in margin analysis.[70,71] Compared to TP53, eIF4E overexpression is specific to tumor cells, and is not overexpressed in premalignant lesions. These molecular changes can be present prior to the appearance of histopathologically positive cancer cells. Multiple studies have verified the presence of these markers at the margin as independent predictors of local recurrence despite histologically negative margins. [70,71] Molecular markers are not limited to genetic mutations and can include microsatellite alterations, copy number alterations (CNAs), or epigenetic changes. Microsatellites refer to repetitive unstable segments in the genome that are susceptible to mutations and have been thoroughly investigated to play an important part in tumorigenesis. CNAs refer to the change in number of copies of certain gene segments. Both types of alterations have been investigated in histologically negative margins and when present have an associated increased risk of locoregional recurrence.[63] Despite the promise of these technologies, these genetic alterations are nonspecific and are difficult to apply in the real-time intraoperative setting where immediate margin analysis is required.

Optical Imaging

One of the main limitations to molecular margin analysis is the feasibility of real-time intraoperative use for optimal surgical resection. On the contrary, optical imaging offers a real-time solution to existing challenges in oncologic resection and margin interpretation. In vivo analysis of tumor margins using optical imaging may direct surgeons to better resect a tumor. Ex vivo analysis can highlight areas suspicious for close or positive margins, and direct intraoperative decision-making.

Optical coherence tomography (OCT) identifies microstructural changes in tissue by scanning a near-infrared (NIR) spectrum optical beam and measuring backscattered/reflected light. The mechanics of the technology is like the scattering of sound by ultrasound.[72] This technology enables the production of high-resolution cross-sectional images of resected tumor tissue.[73] In practice, resected head and neck tumors can be scanned utilizing real-time OCT technology to detect architectural changes indicating tumor presence at surgical margins (**Fig. 3**).[72,73] A study by Badhey and colleagues[73] sought to evaluate margins in oral cavity and oropharyngeal tumor utilizing this technology. Sixty-nine specimens from 2018 to 2019 underwent immediate OCT and subsequent standard of care permanent histology. This study suggested that microstructural changes in benign versus cancerous tissue detected by OCT correlated with histopathologic changes on permanent histology.

While OCT relies on tissue microstructure, fluorescence provides biochemical and molecular information. Fluorescence indicates the process of absorbing shorter wavelength light and the subsequent spontaneous emission of red-shifted light (NIR 700–900 nm light).[74] This light is then detected by a camera and portrayed either on a monitor or through an eyepiece. Light at this wavelength minimizes background nose, has deeper penetration, and is safe with a relatively long half-life. Well-studied fluorophores in this NIR range include the cyanine class of dyes: indocyanine green (ICG), ZW800-1, and IRDye800-CW. ICG typically binds proteins in the plasma and can extravasate and bind to tumor regions using the enhanced permeability and retention effect.[74,75] To further increase the specificity, the fluorophores can be conjugated to bind cancer-specific antibodies.[76] Current antibodies that serve as conjugates include cetuximab and panitumumab (epidermal growth factor receptor inhibitors) and bevacizumab

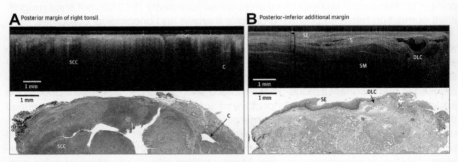

Fig. 3. Representative comparison of images for patient A. Comparison is shown between wide-field optical coherence tomography and permanent histology of invasive, moderately differentiated squamous cell carcinoma (SCC, p16 negative) with lymphatic invasion. (*A*) The posterior margin of the right tonsil is shown, with wide-field optical coherence tomography in the top panel showing SCC as an area with decreased light penetrance depth compared with the adjacent normal tonsillar lymphatic tissue. In the bottom panel, a hematoxylin and eosin slide from the corresponding region is shown. A crypt (C) is also seen on the right side of the image. (*B*) The posterior-inferior additional margin is shown, with wide-field optical coherence tomography in the top panel showing squamous epithelium (SE), submucosal layer (S), and skeletal muscle (SM). In the bottom panel, a hematoxylin and eosin slide from corresponding region is shown. A dilated lymphatic channel (DLC) is also seen on the right side of the image. (*From* Badhey AK, Schwarz JS, Laitman BM, et al. Intraoperative Use of Wide-Field Optical Coherence Tomography to Evaluate Tissue Microstructure in the Oral Cavity and Oropharynx. JAMA Otolaryngol Head Neck Surg.2023;149(1):71–78. https://doi.org/10.1001/jamaoto.2022.3763.)

(targeting vascular endothelial growth factor). ICG has the limitation of being nonspecific and difficult to conjugate giving rise to IRDye800-CW as the most common fluorophore under investigation. IRDye800-CW conjugated to bevacizumab, cetuximab, and panitumumab has been the subject of clinical trials in head and neck cancer surgery.[77] The first phase 1 clinical study involving human subjects by Rosenthal and colleagues[78] used a dose escalation of IRDye800-CW conjugated to cetuximab in 12 patients undergoing surgery for head and neck cancer. This study provided feasibility of fluorescently labeled antibodies with no grade 2 or above adverse events and a 5.2 tumor to background ratio. De Boer and colleagues[77] further demonstrated the accuracy of tumor detection using the cetuximab IRDye800-CW conjugate. Samples from 9 patients with HNSCC injected with IRDye800-CW demonstrated the ability of in vivo fluorescence IHC to specifically detect tumor cells within 1 mm of tumor edge ($P<.001$).

More recently IRDye800-CW conjugated to panitumumab has been investigated for real-time intraoperative tumor margin assessment. Gao and colleagues[79] studied 21 patients with HSNCC undergoing surgery receiving panitumumab-IRDye-800CW at various dosages. Fluorescence correlated to tumor location with sensitives and specificities of greater than 89% with an in vivo tumor to background ratio of 2 to 3. This technique allowed for the creation of a fluorescent map distinguishing the distance from tumor edge to specimen periphery. This optical map can ultimately guide margin sampling.[80] Ex vivo optical specimen mapping can identify areas of highest fluorescence intensity peaks correlating with the closest histopathologic margin 100% of the time.[81,82] These fluorescence intensity peaks can be used as a 'sentinel margin,' where the highest peak correlates with the closest margin (**Fig. 4**). These studies highlight the ability of this technology to (1) detect tumor margins intraoperatively to enhance surgical resection and to (2) improve margin sampling after tumor resection. One of the main limitations of this protocol is that the patient must receive an infusion prior to surgery. In addition, the penetration depth of NIR fluorescence is approximately 5 mm making assessment of complex large head and neck tumors difficult. Though this depth is convenient in assessing margins in head and neck cancer, with close margins traditionally being evaluated at less than 5 mm from the specimen edge. [74] As with any technology, additional limitations include standardization of protocol, Food and Drug Administration approval to maintain standards of safety, and transferability to other institutions.

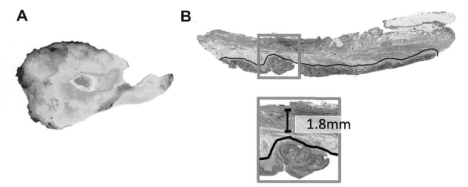

Fig. 4. Correlation of peak fluorescence and histopathologic analysis after administration of tumor-specific contrast agent (panitumumab-IRDye800CW). (*A*) A bright-field of a head and neck squamous cell carcinoma specimen with identified highest fluorescence intensity peaks (*red color*). (*B*) Hematoxylin and eosin (H&E) slide correlative of highest fluorescence intensity peak in panel A with tumor delineated by black line to assess margin distance.

Spectroscopy

Molecular targets encompass one type of optical imaging. Alternative methods of optical imaging rely on inherent fluorescent, vibrational, or rotational properties of tumor versus normal cells.[63] Spectroscopy depends on these properties to scatter light. In this setting, scattered light can be detected to differentiate normal versus malignant tissue at the margin of the specimen. Spectroscopy techniques are limited by resolution due to background fluorescence and poor penetration making it difficult to assess negative results. A study by Hoesli and colleagues[83] utilized Raman spectroscopy, which analyzes the intrinsic vibrational characteristics of molecules, to discriminate between malignant head and neck and benign samples. The investigators found that amongst 42 tumor samples and 42 adjacent normal controls, Raman spectroscopy had a sensitivity and specificity of 88.1% and 95.2% in discriminating between malignant and nonmalignant tissue. These results can offer real-time margin analysis and provide specificity and sensitivity like FSA. Further studies validating the use of Raman spectroscopy have indicated a mean difference of margin length between that depicted by spectroscopy versus histopathologic examination of only 0.17 mm.[84] This exciting technology may be able to mitigate some of the labor-intensive challenges of molecular markers and provide real-time actionable analysis for margin management in head and neck cancer.

Artificial Intelligence

An advanced technique related to spectroscopy is hyperspectral imaging (HSI). HSI combines spectroscopy and digital imaging.[85] This technique provides both spectral and spatial information. The benefit of this technology in margin analysis is that it can demarcate the tumor periphery in a 3D space based on spectral information.[85] Given the large amount of processed spectral data displayed, interpretation can be challenging. Artificial intelligence and machine learning (ML) algorithms can aid in processing and automation of HSI for margin detection and quantification.[86–90] ML uses data at multiple levels to imitate intelligent human behavior thereby improving performance over time. Pertzborn and colleagues[86] investigated the combination of HSI and ML for tumor classification and segmentation using 23 unstained tissue sections from 7 patients with oral cavity squamous cell carcinoma. This was compared to traditional FSA of margins. This technology was able to delineate tumor margins with an accuracy of 76% and a specificity of 89%, introducing HIS and ML as a possible tool for margin analysis. Importantly, the processing time for margin analysis was around 10 minutes per slice, proving equivalent, if not superior, to FSA. Although this technology is still far from maturity, it provides exciting new possibilities in margin classification and segmentation. HSI and ML can go beyond binary classification of tumor margins and hypothetically detect molecular signatures to further enrich the field of margin analysis.[86]

Need for a Novel Metric for Intraoperative Head and Neck Cancer Surgery Interventions

Ultimately, investigators will need to demonstrate clinical value for novel intraoperative technology and real-time intraoperative margin assessment. Clinical trials require sufficient statistical power to detect differences between groups that are of clinical interest. For the aforementioned novel techniques, downstream outcomes such as overall survival and local control would require hundreds of patients randomized in a prospective clinical trial. Demonstrating a decrease in positive surgical margins using novel technology is challenging in a prospective surgical clinical trial. For example, if one were to conduct a clinical trial examining a novel intraoperative technology for locally advanced oral cavity cancer (cT3-T4 baseline positive surgical margin rate of 18%)[91] and wanted

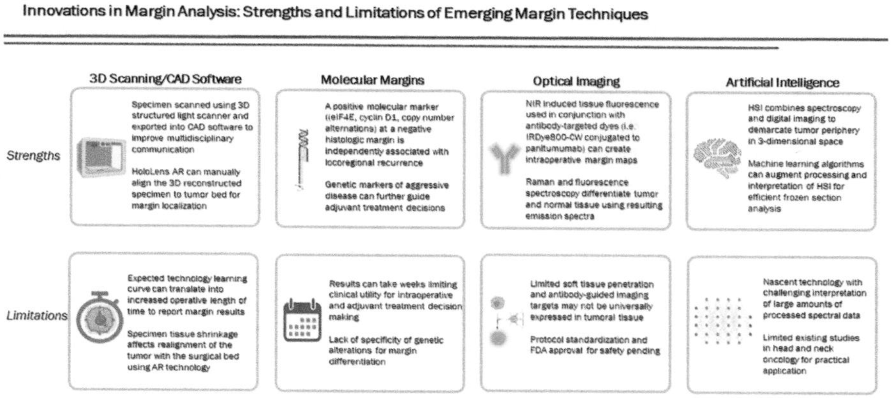

Innovations in Margin Analysis: Strengths and Limitations of Emerging Margin Techniques

Fig. 5. Strengths and limitations of novel margin analysis techniques. AR, augmented reality; CAD, computer-aided design; eIF4E, eukaryotic translocation initiation factor 4E; HIS, hyperspectral imaging.

to demonstrate that the novel technology improved surgical margins to the positive surgical margin rate of early stage oral cavity cancer (cT1-T2 baseline positive surgical margin rate of 8%),[92] this would require 176 patients per arm (power = 0.80, type 1 error probability 0.05). A clinical trial designed with a primary endpoint of margin distance may still be clinically relevant and more feasible to complete. Finally, a validated novel endpoint that incorporates initial margin status on FSA, approach to margins, and a surgeon's perception of case difficulty could also be valuable.

SUMMARY

Obtaining a negative surgical margin is critical to oncological success in patients with head and neck cancer. Currently, surgeons resect tumor with a cuff of perceived normal tissue based on manual palpation and visualization. There exists no clear consensus on the definition of a negative or close margin with most studies citing a margin less than 5 mm as being close. This definition does not apply to all subsites as smaller margins for early laryngeal tumors and HPV-mediated oropharyngeal tumors likely provide adequate local control. Margins are either obtained from specimen or tumor bed and FSA is used to direct further decisions regarding reresection. Sampling error and localization of margins for reresection are established limitations of the current margin analysis system. Emerging technologies to optimize margin management include novel 3D scanning technology and CAD software with AR to enhance intraoperative communication between the surgeon and the pathologist and fluorescence-guided surgery. Molecular margins, optical imaging, and artificial intelligence show promise in further enhancing oncologic surgical resection and accurate margin sampling to guide multidisciplinary oncologic management. A summary of strengths and limitations of described margin analysis techniques is highlighted in **Fig. 5**.

CLINICS CARE POINTS

Pearls
- Current intraoperative margin assessment technique includes FSA to allow for real-time margin assessment and reresection if positive.

- Tumor bed margins improve accuracy of margin assessment and improve local control compared to specimen-based margins.
- Sampling, relocalization, and interpretive errors are known challenges in FSA.
- Innovation in margin analysis includes enhanced pathologist-surgeon interaction using 3D scanning technology and CAD software with AR, molecular margins, optical imaging, spectroscopy, and artificial intelligence.

DISCLOSURE

The authors have nothing to disclose.

REFERENCES

1. Loree TR, Strong EW. Significance of positive margins in oral cavity squamous carcinoma. Am J Surg 1990;160(4):410–4.
2. Jesse RH, Sugarbaker EV. Squamous cell carcinoma of the oropharynx: why we fail. Am J Surg 1976;132(4):435–8.
3. Bernier J, Cooper JS, Pajak TF, et al. Defining risk levels in locally advanced head and neck cancers: a comparative analysis of concurrent postoperative radiation plus chemotherapy trials of the EORTC (#22931) and RTOG (# 9501). Head Neck 2005;27(10):843–50.
4. Cooper JS, Pajak TF, Forastiere AA, et al. Postoperative concurrent radiotherapy and chemotherapy for high-risk squamous-cell carcinoma of the head and neck. N Engl J Med 2004;350(19):1937–44.
5. NCCN. National comprehensive cancer network clinical practice guidelines in oncology (nccn guidelines) head and neck cancers. 2024. Available at: www.nccn.org. [Accessed 26 January 2024].
6. Looser KG, Shah JP, Strong EW. The significance of "positive" margins in surgically resected epidermoid carcinomas. Head Neck Surg Nov-Dec 1978;1(2):107–11.
7. Singh A, Mishra A, Singhvi H, et al. Optimum surgical margins in squamous cell carcinoma of the oral tongue: Is the current definition adequate? Oral Oncol 2020;111:104938.
8. Zanoni DK, Migliacci JC, Xu B, et al. A proposal to redefine close surgical margins in squamous cell carcinoma of the oral tongue. JAMA Otolaryngol Head Neck Surg 2017;143(6):555–60.
9. Bulbul MG, Zenga J, Tarabichi O, et al. Margin practices in oral cavity cancer resections: survey of american head and neck society members. Laryngoscope 2021;131(4):782–7.
10. Kurita H, Nakanishi Y, Nishizawa R, et al. Impact of different surgical margin conditions on local recurrence of oral squamous cell carcinoma. Oral Oncol 2010;46(11):814–7.
11. Sopka DM, Li T, Lango MN, et al. Dysplasia at the margin? Investigating the case for subsequent therapy in 'low-risk' squamous cell carcinoma of the oral tongue. Oral Oncol 2013;49(11):1083–7.
12. Al-Sarraf M, Pajak TF, Byhardt RW, et al. Postoperative radiotherapy with concurrent cisplatin appears to improve locoregional control of advanced, resectable head and neck cancers: RTOG 88-24. Int J Radiat Oncol Biol Phys 1997;37(4):777–82.

13. Urken ML, Yun J, Saturno MP, et al. Frozen section analysis in head and neck surgical pathology: a narrative review of the past, present, and future of intraoperative pathologic consultation. Oral Oncol 2023;143:106445.

14. Weinstock YE, Alava I 3rd, Dierks EJ. Pitfalls in determining head and neck surgical margins. Oral Maxillofac Surg Clin North Am 2014;26(2):151–62.

15. Wolf GT, Winter W, Bellile E, et al. Histologic pattern of invasion and epithelial-mesenchymal phenotype predict prognosis in squamous carcinoma of the head and neck. Oral Oncol 2018;87:29–35.

16. Mohamed S, Jawad H, Sullivan RO, et al. Significance of worst pattern of invasion-5 in early-stage oral cavity squamous cell carcinoma. Head Neck Pathol 2023;17(3):679–87.

17. Köhler HF, Vartanian JG, Pinto CAL, et al. The impact of worst pattern of invasion on the extension of surgical margins in oral squamous cell carcinoma. Head Neck 2022;44(3):691–7.

18. Meier JD, Oliver DA, Varvares MA. Surgical margin determination in head and neck oncology: current clinical practice. The results of an International American Head and Neck Society Member Survey. Head Neck 2005;27(11):952–8.

19. Byers RM, Bland KI, Borlase B, et al. The prognostic and therapeutic value of frozen section determinations in the surgical treatment of squamous carcinoma of the head and neck. Am J Surg 1978;136(4):525–8.

20. DiNardo LJ, Lin J, Karageorge LS, et al. Accuracy, utility, and cost of frozen section margins in head and neck cancer surgery. Laryngoscope 2000;110(10 Pt 1): 1773–6.

21. Gandour-Edwards RF, Donald PJ, Lie JT. Clinical utility of intraoperative frozen section diagnosis in head and neck surgery: a quality assurance perspective. Head Neck Sep-Oct 1993;15(5):373–6.

22. Ikemura K, Ohya R. The accuracy and usefulness of frozen-section diagnosis. Head Neck Jul-Aug 1990;12(4):298–302.

23. Remsen KA, Lucente FE, Biller HF. Reliability of frozen section diagnosis in head and neck neoplasms. Laryngoscope 1984;94(4):519–24.

24. Du E, Ow TJ, Lo YT, et al. Refining the utility and role of Frozen section in head and neck squamous cell carcinoma resection. Laryngoscope 2016;126(8): 1768–75.

25. Olson SM, Hussaini M, Lewis JS Jr. Frozen section analysis of margins for head and neck tumor resections: reduction of sampling errors with a third histologic level. Mod Pathol 2011;24(5):665–70.

26. Hinni ML, Ferlito A, Brandwein-Gensler MS, et al. Surgical margins in head and neck cancer: a contemporary review. Head Neck 2013;35(9):1362–70.

27. Maxwell JH, Thompson LD, Brandwein-Gensler MS, et al. Early oral tongue squamous cell carcinoma: sampling of margins from tumor bed and worse local control. JAMA Otolaryngol Head Neck Surg 2015;141(12):1104–10.

28. Amit M, Na'ara S, Leider-Trejo L, et al. Improving the rate of negative margins after surgery for oral cavity squamous cell carcinoma: A prospective randomized controlled study. Head Neck 2016;38(Suppl 1):E1803–9.

29. Datta S, Mishra A, Chaturvedi P, et al. Frozen section is not cost beneficial for the assessment of margins in oral cancer. Indian J Cancer Jan-Mar 2019;56(1): 19–23.

30. Mair M, Nair D, Nair S, et al. Intraoperative gross examination vs frozen section for achievement of adequate margin in oral cancer surgery. Oral Surg Oral Med Oral Pathol Oral Radiol 2017;123(5):544–9.

31. Nentwig K, Unterhuber T, Wolff KD, et al. The impact of intraoperative frozen section analysis on final resection margin status, recurrence, and patient outcome with oral squamous cell carcinoma. Clin Oral Investig 2021;25(12):6769–77.

32. Patel RS, Goldstein DP, Guillemaud J, et al. Impact of positive frozen section microscopic tumor cut-through revised to negative on oral carcinoma control and survival rates. Head Neck 2010;32(11):1444–51.

33. Szewczyk M, Golusinski W, Pazdrowski J, et al. Positive fresh frozen section margins as an adverse independent prognostic factor for local recurrence in oral cancer patients. Laryngoscope 2018;128(5):1093–8.

34. Ettl T, El-Gindi A, Hautmann M, et al. Positive frozen section margins predict local recurrence in R0-resected squamous cell carcinoma of the head and neck. Oral Oncol 2016;55:17–23.

35. Bulbul MG, Tarabichi O, Sethi RK, et al. Does clearance of positive margins improve local control in oral cavity cancer? a meta-analysis. Otolaryngol Head Neck Surg 2019;161(2):235–44.

36. Tassone P, Savard C, Topf MC, et al. Association of positive initial margins with survival among patients with squamous cell carcinoma treated with total laryngectomy. JAMA Otolaryngol Head Neck Surg 2018;144(11):1030–6.

37. Zhang L, Judd RT, Zhao S, et al. Immediate resection of positive margins improves local control in oral tongue cancer. Oral Oncol 2023;141:106402.

38. Prasad K, Sharma R, Habib D, et al. How often is cancer present in oral cavity re-resections after initial positive margins? Laryngoscope 2024;134(2):717–24.

39. Nakayama M, Holsinger C, Okamoto M, et al. Clinicopathological analyses of fifty supracricoid laryngectomized specimens: evidence base supporting minimal margins. ORL J Otorhinolaryngol Relat Spec 2009;71(6):305–11.

40. Sigston E, de Mones E, Babin E, et al. Early-stage glottic cancer: oncological results and margins in laser cordectomy. Arch Otolaryngol Head Neck Surg 2006;132(2):147–52.

41. Hartl DM, de Monès E, Hans S, et al. Treatment of early-stage glottic cancer by transoral laser resection. Ann Otol Rhinol Laryngol 2007;116(11):832–6.

42. Brøndbo K, Fridrich K, Boysen M. Laser surgery of T1a glottic carcinomas; significance of resection margins. Eur Arch Oto-Rhino-Laryngol 2007;264(6):627–30.

43. Peretti G, Piazza C, Cocco D, et al. Transoral CO(2) laser treatment for T(is)-T(3) glottic cancer: the University of Brescia experience on 595 patients. Head Neck 2010;32(8):977–83.

44. Pool C, Weaver T, Zhu J, et al. Surgical margin determination in the era of HPV-positive oropharyngeal cancer. Laryngoscope 2021;131(10):E2650–4.

45. Hinni ML, Zarka MA, Hoxworth JM. Margin mapping in transoral surgery for head and neck cancer. Laryngoscope 2013;123(5):1190–8.

46. Tomblinson CM, Fletcher GP, Hu LS, et al. Determination of posterolateral oropharyngeal wall thickness and the potential implications for transoral surgical margins in tonsil cancer. Head Neck 2021;43(7):2185–92.

47. Ryan WR, Xu MJ, Ochoa E, et al. Oncologic outcomes of human papillomavirus-associated oropharynx carcinoma treated with surgery alone: A 12-institution study of 344 patients. Cancer 2021;127(17):3092–106.

48. Holcomb AJ, Richmon JD. Surgical margins in a single-modality transoral robotic surgery: A conundrum-Reply. Head Neck 2021;43(10):3219–21.

49. Iyer NG, Dogan S, Palmer F, et al. Detailed analysis of clinicopathologic factors demonstrate distinct difference in outcome and prognostic factors between

surgically treated hpv-positive and negative oropharyngeal cancer. Ann Surg Oncol 2015;22(13):4411–21.

50. Kerawala CJ, Ong TK. Relocating the site of frozen sections–is there room for improvement? Head Neck 2001;23(3):230–2.

51. Banoub RG, Crippen MM, Fiorella MA, et al. Variance in 3D anatomic localization of surgical margins based on conventional margin labeling in head and neck squamous cell carcinoma. Oral Oncol 2023;139:106360.

52. Coutu B, Ryan E, Christensen D, et al. Positive margins matter regardless of subsequent resection findings. Oral Oncol 2022;128:105850.

53. Tasche KK, Buchakjian MR, Pagedar NA, et al. Definition of "close margin" in oral cancer surgery and association of margin distance with local recurrence rate. JAMA Otolaryngol Head Neck Surg 2017;143(12):1166–72.

54. Buchakjian MR, Tasche KK, Robinson RA, et al. Association of main specimen and tumor bed margin status with local recurrence and survival in oral cancer surgery. JAMA Otolaryngol Head Neck Surg 2016;142(12):1191–8.

55. Black C, Marotti J, Zarovnaya E, et al. Critical evaluation of frozen section margins in head and neck cancer resections. Cancer 2006;107(12):2792–800.

56. Brandwein-Weber M, Urken ML, Topf MC, et al. Radical shift in the communication paradigm in head and neck frozen section analysis: Intraoperative three-dimensional specimen scanning. Head Neck 2023;45(1):7–9.

57. Sharif KF, Prasad K, Miller A, et al. Enhanced intraoperative communication of tumor margins using 3d scanning and mapping: the computer-aided design margin. Laryngoscope 2023;133(8):1914–8.

58. Sharif KF, Lewis JS Jr, Ely KA, et al. The computer-aided design margin: Ex vivo 3D specimen mapping to improve communication between surgeons and pathologists. Head Neck 2023;45(1):22–31.

59. Prasad K, Miller A, Sharif K, et al. Augmented-reality surgery to guide head and neck cancer re-resection: a feasibility and accuracy study. Ann Surg Oncol 2023; 30(8):4994–5000.

60. Johnson RE, Sigman JD, Funk GF, et al. Quantification of surgical margin shrinkage in the oral cavity. Head Neck 1997;19(4):281–6.

61. Umstattd LA, Mills JC, Critchlow WA, et al. Shrinkage in oral squamous cell carcinoma: An analysis of tumor and margin measurements in vivo, post-resection, and post-formalin fixation. Am J Otolaryngol Nov-Dec 2017;38(6):660–2.

62. Mistry RC, Qureshi SS, Kumaran C. Post-resection mucosal margin shrinkage in oral cancer: quantification and significance. J Surg Oncol 2005;91(2):131–3.

63. Stepan KO, Li MM, Kang SY, et al. Molecular margins in head and neck cancer: Current techniques and future directions. Oral Oncol 2020;110:104893.

64. Lane DP. Cancer. p53, guardian of the genome. Nature 1992;358(6381):15–6.

65. Agrawal N, Frederick MJ, Pickering CR, et al. Exome sequencing of head and neck squamous cell carcinoma reveals inactivating mutations in NOTCH1. Science 2011;333(6046):1154–7.

66. van Houten VM, Leemans CR, Kummer JA, et al. Molecular diagnosis of surgical margins and local recurrence in head and neck cancer patients: a prospective study. Clin Cancer Res 2004;10(11):3614–20.

67. Pena Murillo C, Huang X, Hills A, et al. The utility of molecular diagnostics to predict recurrence of head and neck carcinoma. Br J Cancer 2012;107(7):1138–43.

68. Pierssens D, Borgemeester MC, van der Heijden SJH, et al. Chromosome instability in tumor resection margins of primary OSCC is a predictor of local recurrence. Oral Oncol 2017;66:14–21.

69. Nathan CO, Sanders K, Abreo FW, et al. Correlation of p53 and the proto-oncogene eIF4E in larynx cancers: prognostic implications. Cancer Res 2000; 60(13):3599–604.

70. Singh J, Jayaraj R, Baxi S, et al. Immunohistochemical expression levels of p53 and eIF4E markers in histologically negative surgical margins, and their association with the clinical outcome of patients with head and neck squamous cell carcinoma. Mol Clin Oncol 2016;4(2):166–72.

71. Sakashita T, Homma A, Suzuki S, et al. Prognostic value of cyclin D1 expression in tumor-free surgical margins in head and neck squamous cell carcinomas. Acta Otolaryngol 2013;133(9):984–91.

72. Yuan S, Roney CA, Wierwille J, et al. Co-registered optical coherence tomography and ffluorescence molecular imaging for simultaneous morphological and molecular imaging. Phys Med Biol 2010;55(1):191–206.

73. Badhey AK, Schwarz JS, Laitman BM, et al. Intraoperative use of wide-field optical coherence tomography to evaluate tissue microstructure in the oral cavity and oropharynx. JAMA Otolaryngol Head Neck Surg 2023;149(1):71–8.

74. Lee YJ, Krishnan G, Nishio N, et al. Intraoperative fluorescence-guided surgery in head and neck squamous cell carcinoma. Laryngoscope 2021;131(3):529–34.

75. Zhang RR, Schroeder AB, Grudzinski JJ, et al. Beyond the margins: real-time detection of cancer using targeted fluorophores. Nat Rev Clin Oncol 2017; 14(6):347–64.

76. Iqbal H, Pan Q. Image guided surgery in the management of head and neck cancer. Oral Oncol 2016;57:32–9.

77. de Boer E, Warram JM, Tucker MD, et al. In vivo fluorescence immunohistochemistry: localization of fluorescently labeled cetuximab in squamous cell carcinomas. Sci Rep 2015;5:10169.

78. Rosenthal EL, Warram JM, de Boer E, et al. Safety and tumor specificity of cetuximab-irdye800 for surgical navigation in head and neck cancer. Clin Cancer Res 2015;21(16):3658–66.

79. Gao RW, Teraphongphom NT, van den Berg NS, et al. Determination of tumor margins with surgical specimen mapping using near-infrared fluorescence. Cancer Res 2018;78(17):5144–54.

80. van Keulen S, van den Berg NS, Nishio N, et al. Rapid, non-invasive fluorescence margin assessment: Optical specimen mapping in oral squamous cell carcinoma. Oral Oncol 2019;88:58–65.

81. van Keulen S, Nishio N, Birkeland A, et al. The sentinel margin: intraoperative ex vivo specimen mapping using relative fluorescence intensity. Clin Cancer Res 2019;25(15):4656–62.

82. Fakurnejad S, Krishnan G, van Keulen S, et al. Intraoperative molecular imaging for ex vivo assessment of peripheral margins in oral squamous cell carcinoma. Front Oncol 2019;9:1476.

83. Hoesli RC, Orringer DA, McHugh JB, et al. Coherent raman scattering microscopy for evaluation of head and neck carcinoma. Otolaryngol Head Neck Surg 2017;157(3):448–53.

84. Aaboubout Y, Nunes Soares MR, Bakker Schut TC, et al. Intraoperative assessment of resection margins by Raman spectroscopy to guide oral cancer surgery. Analyst 2023;148(17):4116–26.

85. Lu G, Fei B. Medical hyperspectral imaging: a review. J Biomed Opt 2014;19(1): 10901.

86. Pertzborn D, Nguyen HN, Hüttmann K, et al. Intraoperative assessment of tumor margins in tissue sections with hyperspectral imaging and machine learning. Cancers (Basel) 2022;15(1). https://doi.org/10.3390/cancers15010213.
87. Halicek M, Fabelo H, Ortega S, et al. Hyperspectral imaging for head and neck cancer detection: specular glare and variance of the tumor margin in surgical specimens. J Med Imaging 2019;6(3):035004.
88. Halicek M, Dormer JD, Little JV, et al. Hyperspectral imaging of head and neck squamous cell carcinoma for cancer margin detection in surgical specimens from 102 patients using deep learning. Cancers (Basel) 2019;11(9). https://doi.org/10.3390/cancers11091367.
89. Lu G, Little JV, Wang X, et al. Detection of head and neck cancer in surgical specimens using quantitative hyperspectral imaging. Clin Cancer Res 2017;23(18): 5426–36.
90. Loperfido A, Celebrini A, Marzetti A, et al. Current role of artificial intelligence in head and neck cancer surgery: a systematic review of literature. Explor Target Antitumor Ther 2023;4(5):933–40.
91. Prasad K, Topf MC, Clookey S, et al. Trends in positive surgical margins in cT3-T4 oral cavity squamous cell carcinoma. Otolaryngol Head Neck Surg 2023;169(5): 1200–7.
92. Robinson EM, Lam AS, Solomon I, et al. Trends in positive surgical margins in ct1-t2 oral cavity squamous cell carcinoma. Laryngoscope 2022;132(10):1962–70.

Disparities in Care for Patients with Head and Neck Cancer

Alejandro R. Marrero-Gonzalez, BS[a],
Evan M. Graboyes, MD, MPH[a,b,c],*

KEYWORDS

- Cancer disparities • Head and neck cancer • Social determinants of health
- Cancer care

KEY POINTS

- Disparities in head and neck cancer are shaped by social determinants of health and factors that influence multiple levels of health behavior.
- Significant disparities in head and neck cancer incidence and survival exist among racial groups; Black patients have a higher mortality rate compared with White patients.
- Lower socioeconomic status and lack of health insurance are associated with delays in diagnosis and advanced stage at diagnosis.
- Race, ethnicity, insurance status, and socioeconomic factors influence timely cancer care and guideline adherence.

INTRODUCTION

For patients with head and neck squamous cell carcinoma (HNSCC) disparities exist for members of certain racial and ethnic, gender, socioeconomic, or geographic groups.[1,2] These disparities are well documented and exist along the cancer continuum, from risk factors and incidence through treatment and survivorship (**Fig. 1**).[3] For example, the incidence of human papillomavirus (HPV)-negative pharyngeal and laryngeal SCC is higher among non-Hispanic Black patients than among non-Hispanic White patients.[4] Disparities in timely care exist for patients with HNSCC, as patients with Medicaid insurance are 2 times more likely to experience a delay in treatment initiation relative to patients with commercial insurance.[5] Profound racial

[a] Department of Otolaryngology–Head & Neck Surgery, Medical University of South Carolina, 135 Rutledge Avenue, MSC 550, Charleston, SC 29425, USA; [b] Department of Public Health Sciences, Medical University of South Carolina, Charleston, SC, USA; [c] Hollings Cancer Center, Medical University of South Carolina, Charleston, SC, USA
* Corresponding author. Department of Otolaryngology - Head & Neck Surgery, Medical University of South Carolina, 135 Rytledge Avenue, MSC 550, Charleston, SC 29425.
E-mail address: graboyes@musc.edu

Surg Oncol Clin N Am 33 (2024) 669–681
https://doi.org/10.1016/j.soc.2024.04.010
surgonc.theclinics.com

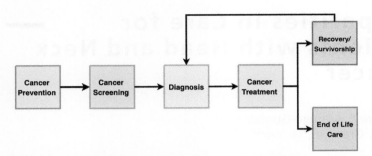

Fig. 1. Cancer care continuum domains. (*From* National Cancer Institute. Cancer Control Continuum. Division of Cancer Control & Population Sciences, National Cancer Institute, National Institutes of Health. 2023. https://cancercontrol.cancer.gov/about-dccps/about-cc/cancer-control-continuum.)

differences in survival also exist. Black patients with HNSCC are 72% more likely to die than their White counterparts.[6] In fact, of all cancer types, HNSCC has the third largest difference in mortality between White and Black patients.[6] Furthermore, geographic location is important; patients with HNSCC living in rural areas have 11% increased mortality relative to patients from urban areas.[7]

In this article, we explore disparities along the cancer continuum by demographic factors (race, ethnicity, gender, socioeconomic status (SES), insurance, and geography) for patients with HNSCC in the United States. After introducing key disparity-related terminology and highlighting conceptual frameworks for understanding cancer disparities, we review disparities in HNSCC incidence, severity, treatment timeliness, guideline adherence, and oncologic outcomes. Toward the end of this article, we review possible interventions to address these disparities.

Background: Terminology and Conceptual Frameworks

Careful use of vocabulary promotes clarity, sensitivity, and accuracy when communicating with patients, caregivers, clinicians, and scientific colleagues.[8] To provide an important foundation and ensure that words are used precisely and accurately, we start the article by explaining key disparity-related terminology (**Table 1**).[7–13] Although the structure of the article follows descriptions of observed disparities for certain minoritized groups, we recognize the reductionist nature of focusing on one single attribute (eg, race or insurance) when many risk factors covary in marginalized populations (eg, no health insurance and lower income).

Health behavior theory suggests our actions are influenced by a variety of sources. Often, we consider the determinants of behavior at an individual level, but health-related behavior is also shaped by factors at the interpersonal (eg, relationship with a spouse or caregiver), institutional (eg, hospital resources), community (eg, access to health care resources), and public policy levels (eg, laws).[14] Collectively, these determinants of behavior across multiple levels of influence, or multilevel determinants, influence cancer risk and outcomes.[15] The socioecological framework is widely used to understand the multilevel determinants contributing to health and health disparities (**Fig. 2**). The social–ecological framework recognizes that personal choices and genetics do not solely determine individual health outcomes. Rather, health (and differences in health between groups) is shaped and profoundly influenced by the broader socioecological context. Multilevel consideration within this framework, such as assessing the impact of community-level measures of social disadvantage, is important to comprehensively understand and address cancer disparities.

Table 1
Definitions of important disparity-related vocabulary terms

Terms	Definition	Example
Difference	Variation in health outcome between 2 groups	Older adults have higher mortality than younger adults.
Disparity	A health difference that adversely affects disadvantaged populations based on one or more health outcomes.[9]	Black patients with HNSCC have worse survival than White patients with HNSCC.
Inequity	A systematic and unjust difference in health status or the distribution of health resources between different population groups arising from social determinants of health.[63] Health inequities are unfair and could be reduced through changes in government policies.	Black patients with HNSCC face barriers to accessing timely care, such as limited access to screening, diagnostic services, or treatment options, while White patients have more access to these resources.
Race	A social construct categorizing individuals into groups based on physical characteristics, such as skin color, with no biological basis but significant social implications.[8]	White, Black, Asian
Ethnicity	A shared cultural identity, including common language, traditions, and history, often linked to a particular geographic or national origin and can be a component of a person's identity.[8]	Hispanic, Non-Hispanic
Ancestry	A biological (ie, genetic) construct that refers to a person's country or region of origin or an individual's lineage of descent.[8]	African, European, and Native American
Gender	The socially constructed norms, behaviors, and roles associated with being a woman, man, girl, or boy, as well as relationships with each other.[7]	Cisgender (cis man, cis women), nonbinary, agender, gender-fluid
Sex	A biological classification based on physical, genetic, reproductive, and physiologic features.[10]	Male, female, or intersex
Social Determinants of Health	The conditions in which people are born, grow up, live, work and age that affect health.[11] Social determinants of health are not intrinsically better or worse.	Education, transportation, job opportunities, access to nutritious food
Health-related Social Risk	An individual-level adverse social determinant of health (ie, an individual-level social attribute or exposure that increases a person's likelihood of poor health).[12]	Food insecurity, transportation problems, housing instability
Health-related Social Need	A health-related social risk for which an individual expresses a preference and priority for having addressed.[13]	An individual requests food assistance because of lack of food

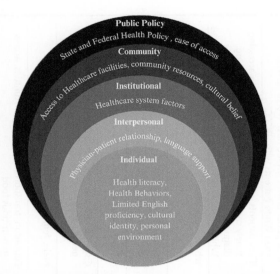

Fig. 2. Socioecological framework applied to health care. (*From* Batool S, Burks CA, Bergmark RW. Healthcare Disparities in Otolaryngology. Curr Otorhinolaryngol Rep. Jun 8 2023:1-14. https://doi.org/10.1007/s40136-023-00459-0.)

There is growing recognition that the social determinants of health (SDOH), the conditions in which people are born, grow up, work, live, and age are key factors in shaping health. These SDOH, which are not intrinsically positive or negative, include things such as housing, transportation, education, job opportunities, and access to nutritious food (**Fig. 3**).[16] For clinicians providing care to patients with HNSCC in a clinic, hospital, or cancer center, the perspective on SDOH is one that is decidedly "downstream" (ie, at the point of care delivery). As recognition that improving

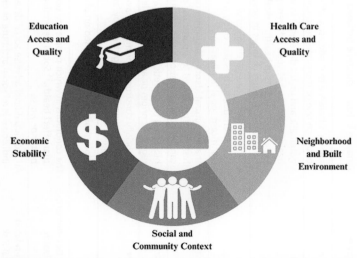

Fig. 3. Healthy People 2030, U.S. Department of Health and Human Services, Office of Disease Prevention and Health Promotion. Retrieved 16 May 2024, from https://health.gov/healthypeople/objectives-and-data/social-determinants-health.

outcomes and equity in oncology care requires integrating social care into health care, health systems are increasingly striving to move upstream (ie, prior to the point of care delivery, such as in the community) in their efforts to address the root causes.[17]

DISPARITIES IN INCIDENCE

Disparities in the incidence of HNSCC occur for certain racial, socioeconomic, and geographic groups. For example, the incidence of HPV-associated oropharyngeal squamous cell cancer is higher in non-Hispanic White male patients compared with Black patients.[18,19] Black patients, on the other hand, have a greater incidence of HPV-negative pharyngeal and laryngeal SCC compared with non-Hispanic White patients.[4] Even though the prevalence of smoking, a risk factor for HPV-negative pharyngeal and laryngeal cancer, is similar among non-Hispanic Black and White patients in the United States, there is a higher incidence of both these cancers among non-Hispanic Black patients.[4,20] Disparities in HNSCC incidence also exist for certain socioeconomic groups. Lower SES has been associated with a lower incidence of HPV-positive HNSCC, but a higher incidence of HNSCC overall.[1,21] Where the patient lives also contributes to disparities in HNSCC incidence, as individuals living in urban areas have a higher incidence of HPV-positive HNSCC relative to those in rural areas.[21]

DISPARITIES IN STAGE AT DIAGNOSIS

HNSCC stage at diagnosis is associated with survival.[22] In fact, differences in stage at presentation between White and Black patients with HNSCC are one of the major determinants of observed racial disparities in survival.[23–25] In a study of 69,186 patients with HNSCC in the National Cancer Database (NCDB), Jassal and Cramer demonstrated that oncologic factors such as stage at presentation accounted for 57.7% of the observed mortally differences between White and Black patients with HNSCC.[23]

Although there are numerous biological and nonbiological factors that affect the stage at diagnosis, access to care and timely care are critically important factors. It is, therefore, not surprising that health insurance coverage is a critical factor influencing the stage at diagnosis for HNSCC.[26] Patients with Medicaid are more likely to present with an advanced tumor classification than patients without Medicaid after adjusting for demographic and tumor characteristics.[27] Patients without health insurance are more likely to present with metastatic disease upon diagnosis.[28] Dental insurance benefits are also related to the stage at diagnosis. In a cohort study of 10,318 patients with oral cavity cancer, Kana and colleagues reported that changes in California Medicaid dental insurance coverage were associated with the diagnosis of stage 0 to II oral cavity cancer after adjusting for potentially confounding demographic factors.[29] In another cohort study with 90,789 patients, Sineshaw and colleagues found that in states with Medicaid expansion through the Affordable Care Act, there was a 2.3% point increase in localized disease at diagnosis when compared with nonexpansion states after adjusting for age, race/ethnicity, and income level.[30] Rurality is also associated with access to care and stage at diagnosis. Patients living in rural areas have fewer providers (including specialists) and longer travel distances,[31] which contribute to the increase in advanced tumor and nodal stage among rural patients with HNSCC upon presentation.[32]

DISPARITIES IN TIMELY CANCER CARE

Timely treatment of HNSCC, from initiation through completion of therapy, is a vital aspect of quality care and correlates with improved oncologic outcomes.[33] Time to treatment initiation (TTI), particularly beyond 60 days, is associated with an increased recurrence rate and worse survival.[5,34] Black patients, Hispanic patients, those with Medicaid insurance, and lower SES are all at an increased risk of delayed treatment initiation in a study using the NCDB.[34] Similar disparities in timely treatment initiation were found in a retrospective cohort study of 956 patients with HNSCC treated at an urban community-based academic center.[5] Distance from treatment is associated with TTI,[35] and even after patients initiate treatment, disparities persist. For example, patients with Medicaid or no health insurance are more likely to experience a prolonged treatment package time (the time from surgery through the completion of radiotherapy) than patients with private/commercial insurance.[36,37]

DISPARITIES IN QUALITY OF CARE/GUIDELINE ADHERENCE

In a study of 69,186 patients with surgically managed HNSCC, Black patients had a lower mean composite score for 5 quality metrics (rate of negative surgical margins, the rate of appropriate adjuvant radiation, the rate of appropriate adjuvant chemoradiation, and timely adjuvant radiation within 6 weeks of surgery) than White patients.[23] For patients with HNSCC, initiation of postoperative radiation therapy (PORT) within 6 weeks of surgery is recommended by the National Comprehensive Cancer Network (NCCN) Clinical Practice Guidelines in Oncology[38] and is the only American College of Surgeons/Commission on Cancer approved quality metric for HNSCC.[39] Black patients, or those with no Medicaid or no health insurance, or those with lower levels of education are less likely to receive guideline-adherent care.[36] The NCCN guidelines also recommend surgery as the preferred treatment of oral cavity SCC. Despite this, Black patients are 13% less likely to receive surgery for oral cavity SCC and more likely to decline surgery when recommended across all subsites of HNSCC.[40,41] In addition, Black patients are more prone to receive treatment at institutions with a higher safety-net burden.[23] Gender-focused studies show women with advanced-stage HNSCC are less likely than men to receive guideline-concordant chemotherapy.[42]

DISPARITIES IN ONCOLOGIC OUTCOMES

Disparities in oncologic outcomes such as survival are observed for racial, ethnic, socioeconomic, insurance, or gender groups. A systematic review/meta-analysis by Russo and colleagues reported Black patients with HNSCC had 27% higher chance of death than White patients with HNSCC (HR 1.27, CI 1.18–1.36) after adjusting for SES.[43] Within the context of therapeutic cooperative group trials where confounders of SES, quality of care, and access to care are minimized, Liu and colleagues found that Black patients with HNSCC had worse survival outcomes than White patients with HNSCC, primarily due to higher rates of locoregional failure.[44]

Interestingly, in a variety of disease settings, despite having a worse risk factor profile, patients with Hispanic ethnicity have improved survival relative to non-Hispanic patients, an epidemiologic phenomenon known as the Hispanic health paradox. These findings hold true for patients with HNSCC. In a study of 45,324 patients with HNSCC in the SEER, Parasher and colleagues found that US-born Hispanic patients with HNSCC have 14% decrease in the odds of mortality (OR 0.86, 95% CI 0.82–0.89) relative to non-Hispanic White patients with HNSCC.[45]

There is extensive literature on the relationship between insurance status, education, and SES and worse survival among patients with HNSCC.[46,47] For example, in a study of 57,920 patients with HNSCC in the SEER database, Pannu and colleagues found that patients with Medicaid or no health insurance were 65% and 55% more likely to die when compared with private insurance, respectively, after adjusting for age at diagnosis, year of diagnosis, county-level poverty percentage, sex, race/ethnicity, marital status, and tumor site.[48] Patients in the lowest income quartile (<\$35,000/y) had a 48% increased mortality relative to patients with higher income, even adjusting coexisting variables (health behaviors, comorbidities, and treatment characteristics).[46] Lower income groups are thought to have worse access to care, present with more advanced-stage disease, and are more likely to experience treatment delays.[49,50] While lower income positively correlates with lower education, these variables are independent risk factors for poor overall survival.[46]

DISPARITIES IN QUALITY OF LIFE

Health-related quality of life (HRQOL) is affected by several factors, including race, geography, and gender. A randomized phase 2 trial found that mean quality of life (QOL) scores were 11.4 points lower in Black patients relative to White patients.[51] The authors suggest that this surprising disparity in QOL within the context of a randomized clinical trial may be due to a range of challenges, such as socioeconomic disadvantages and psychosocial distress that may predominate among Black patients.[51] In a study of the effect of geography on care, 261 patients with HNSCC living in rural areas had a 10 point lower mean HRQOL than those living in urban areas.[52] In a study of gender differences, it was found women with HNSCC had worse QOL than men, with mental health being particularly affected.[53]

DISPARITIES IN CLINICAL TRIAL PARTICIPATION

Equitable patient participation in clinical trials is a pivotal part of improving outcomes for patients with HNSCC.[54] The history of mistrust in the medical system, particularly among Black patients, has been a significant barrier to their participation in clinical trials.[55] This mistrust stems from unethical research practices, such as those exemplified by the Tuskegee Syphilis Study.[55] This mistrust has led to decreased participation of racial and ethnic minorities in clinical trials in several fields of medicine.[55–57] Sauer and colleagues found that Black patients constitute 8% of clinical trial participants despite accounting for 10% of HNSCC cases and that Asian or Pacific Islanders constitute 2% of clinical trial participants despite accounting for 6% of the cases.[58] A positive trend toward equity in representation was observed between 2010 and 2020.[58] However, much room for progress remains. To ensure that clinical trial participants reflect disease demographics and enhance the generalizability of the results, organizations, including the National Institutes of Health and Food and Drug Administration, have implemented policies to improve enrollment of participants from underrepresented racial and ethnic populations into clinical trials.[59] Gender disparities in oncology trial participation are well-documented, with women being underrepresented.[60] Among chemotherapy trials for HNSCC, women account for 17.0% of patients in the trials but 26.2% of patients with HNSCC.[42]

INTERVENTIONS TO ADDRESS DISPARITIES

Key interventions include antitobacco measures, HPV vaccination campaigns, and enhanced access to care through financial assistance, travel support programs, and telehealth services.[61–63] Further, educating non-otolaryngologist health care providers about oral cancer may aid early diagnosis by improving recognition of initial symptoms. Patient navigation-based approaches have also shown promise as a strategy to improve equity in the delivery of guideline-adherent adjuvant radiation therapy for patients with HNSCC. Navigation for Disparities and Untimely Radiation Therapy

(NDURE) is a patient navigation-based intervention targeting barriers to timely PORT at the patient, health care team, and organizational levels through comprehensive measures such as patient education, travel support, and organizational restructuring.[64] In a randomized clinical trial, NDURE showed the potential to enhance equity in timely adjuvant therapy relative to usual care.[65] The difference in delays in initiating guideline-adherent PORT between Black and White patients was 12% in NDURE versus 24% in usual care. The difference in median time to PORT between Black and White patients was 1 day in NDURE versus 10 days in usual care. Patients have many barriers to receiving timely PORT, such as transportation insecurity.[66] Hospitals are prevented from paying for travel for low-income patients due to fear of inducement and kickback rules. Not-for-profit organizations such as the American Cancer Society have developed programs to address this barrier in transportation among patients with cancer.[66] Regarding a more upstream approach, federal and state policies exist for Medicare and Medicaid beneficiaries that offer transportation for nonemergency medical visits.[66]

RESEARCH AGENDA

Historically, disparities research in HNSCC has focused on disparities racial and ethnic groups, by health insurance coverage, SES, and geography.[1] However, emerging data from other tumor types suggest that other factors, sexual orientation and gender identity, and minoritized patients may experience delayed diagnosis and higher recurrence rates.[67] There is a critical need to understand the mechanisms responsible for disparities due to social constructs such as race, ethnicity, and gender, as well as SDOH such as rurality along the care continuum for patients with HNSCC. Both social constructs and SDOH require multilevel inquiry. Using the socioecological framework, we can aim to understand the multilevel determinants contributing to these disparities. To date, the preponderance of research evaluating disparities in HNSCC has been descriptive in nature, identifying associations between individual-level demographic characteristics and outcomes of interest.[1] The research has focused primarily on demographic labels and stayed downstream at the point-of-care delivery. To advance the field and enable equity for patients with HNSCC, future research must characterize the multilevel determinants of the disparities and the downstream social, cultural, and biological pathways that affect human health (and differences in health among groups).[1]

There is a critical lack of research developing and evaluating equity-focused interventions among patients with HNSCC. Tailored treatment strategies should be developed to address the specific needs of underserved populations, reflecting the underlying socioecological model and considering upstream SDOH and health-related social needs. Community-based initiatives and awareness campaigns can help educate at-risk populations about HNSCC risk factors and promote early detection. More research identifying barriers to health care access and advocating for policy changes that ensure equitable access to quality care is critical.

Although race (a social construct) and ancestry (a genetic construct that refers to an individual's region of origin and lineage) are conceptually distinct, additional research is needed to understand the biology underlying ancestry-based differences between groups.[8] For example, studies have begun to explore how ancestry-based differences in DNA damage repair pathways may explain differential treatment effectiveness and disparities in survival among patients with HNSCC.[68] In addition, more studies linking the structural and social drivers to underlying biologic mechanisms will enhance our understanding of disparities and potentially elucidate actionable targets or pathways to enhance equity.

SUMMARY

Profound and pervasive disparities in HNSCC incidence, diagnosis, treatment, outcomes, and participation in clinical trials exist for racial, ethnic, socioeconomic, and geographic groups. Understanding and subsequently addressing these disparities requires a deep understanding of their multilevel determinants and SDOH. Further research is needed to understand the mechanisms driving disparities and develop equity-focused interventions to ensure the best outcomes for all patients with HNSCC.

CLINICS CARE POINTS

Pearls

- Careful use of equity-related vocabulary promotes clarity, sensitivity, and accuracy when communicating with patients, caregivers, clinicians, and scientific colleagues.
- Understanding and addressing profound and pervasive disparities along the cancer care continuum for racial, ethnic, socioeconomic, and geographic groups requires a deep understanding of their multilevel determinants and social determinants of health.
- Patient navigation is an evidence-based intervention to address barriers to care and improve equity among patients with head and neck squamous cell carcinoma.

Pitfalls

- The underrepresentation of black patients and female patients with head and neck squamous cell carcinoma in clinical trials affects the generalizability of clinical trial results, potentially leading to less effective treatment strategies.
- Although integrating social care into healthcare has potential to improve equity in care for patients with head and neck squamous cell carcinoma, clinicians delivering care remain far downstream from the underlying root causes.

DISCLOSURE

The authors have nothing to disclose.

FUNDING

This work was supported by the National Cancer Institute at the National Institutes of Health K08 CA237858 and R01 CA282165 to E.M.G.

REFERENCES

1. Nallani R, Subramanian TL, Ferguson-Square KM, et al. A systematic review of head and neck cancer health disparities: a call for innovative research. Otolaryngology-Head Neck Surg (Tokyo) 2022;166(6):1238–48.
2. Batool S, Burks CA, Bergmark RW. Healthcare disparities in otolaryngology. Curr Otorhinolaryngol Rep 2023;1–14.
3. National Cancer Institute. Cancer control continuum. Division of Cancer Control & Population Sciences, National Cancer Institute, National Institutes of Health. 2023. Available at: https://cancercontrol.cancer.gov/about-dccps/about-cc/cancer-control-continuum.
4. Mazul AL, Chidambaram S, Zevallos JP, et al. Disparities in head and neck cancer incidence and trends by race/ethnicity and sex. Head Neck 2023;45(1):75–84.

5. Liao DZ, Schlecht NF, Rosenblatt G, et al. Association of delayed time to treatment initiation with overall survival and recurrence among patients with head and neck squamous cell carcinoma in an underserved urban population. JAMA otolaryngology– head & neck surgery 2019;145(11):1001–9.

6. Lara OD, Wang Y, Asare A, et al. Pan-cancer clinical and molecular analysis of racial disparities. Cancer 2020;126(4):800–7.

7. World Health Organization, Gender mainstreaming for health managers: a practical approach, 2011, *World Health Organization (WHO)*. Available at: https://www.who.int/publications/i/item/9789241501057.

8. Flanagin A, Frey T, Christiansen SL, et al. Updated guidance on the reporting of race and ethnicity in medical and science journals. JAMA 2021;326(7):621–7.

9. National Institute of Minority and Helath Disparities. Minority Health and Health Disparities: Definitions and Parameters. 2023. Available at: https://www.nimhd.nih.gov/about/strategic-plan/nih-strategic-plan-definitions-and-parameters.html.

10. Bewley S, McCartney M, Meads C, et al. Sex, gender, and medical data. BMJ 2021;372:n735.

11. World Health Organization, Closing the gap in a generation: health equity through action on the social determinants of health, 2008, World Health Organization; Geneva, Switzerland. Available at: https://iris.who.int/bitstream/handle/10665/43943/9789241563703_eng.pdf.

12. Alderwick H, Gottlieb LM. Meanings and misunderstandings: a social determinants of health lexicon for health care systems. Milbank Q 2019;97(2):407–19.

13. Schiavoni KH, Helscel K, Vogeli C, et al. Prevalence of social risk factors and social needs in a Medicaid Accountable Care Organization (ACO). BMC Health Serv Res 2022;22(1):1375.

14. Taplin SH, Anhang Price R, Edwards HM, et al. Introduction: understanding and influencing multilevel factors across the cancer care continuum. JNCI Monographs 2012;2012(44):2–10.

15. US Department of Health. Human Services, Theory at a glance: a guide for health promotion practice. Bethesda, MD: Lulu. com; 2018.

16. Office of Disease Prevention and Health Promotion. Healthy People 2030 - Social Determinants of Health. Available at: https://health.gov/healthypeople/priority-areas/social-determinants-health.

17. National Academies of Sciences, Engineering, and Medicine. 2019. Integrating Social Care into the Delivery of Health Care: Moving Upstream to Improve the Nation's Health. The National Academies Press; Washington, DC. https://doi.org/10.17226/25467.

18. Tota JE, Best AF, Zumsteg ZS, et al. Evolution of the oropharynx cancer epidemic in the United States: moderation of increasing incidence in younger individuals and shift in the burden to older individuals. J Clin Oncol 2019;37(18):1538–46.

19. Damgacioglu H, Sonawane K, Zhu Y, et al. Oropharyngeal cancer incidence and mortality trends in all 50 States in the US, 2001-2017. JAMA Otolaryngol Head Neck Surg 2022;148(2):155–65.

20. Cornelius ME, Loretan CG, Wang TW, et al. Tobacco product use among adults - United States, 2020. MMWR Morb Mortal Wkly Rep 2022;71(11):397–405.

21. Peterson CE, Khosla S, Jefferson GD, et al. Measures of economic advantage associated with HPV-positive head and neck cancers among non-Hispanic black and white males identified through the National Cancer Database. Cancer Epidemiol 2017;48:1–7.

22. Siegel RL, Miller KD, Wagle NS, et al. Cancer statistics, 2023. CA A Cancer J Clin 2023;73(1):17–48.

23. Jassal JS, Cramer JD. Explaining racial disparities in surgically treated head and neck cancer. Laryngoscope 2021;131(5):1053–9.
24. Baliga S, Yildiz VO, Bazan J, et al. Disparities in survival outcomes among racial/ethnic minorities with head and neck squamous cell cancer in the United States. Cancers 2023;15(6).
25. Taylor DB, Osazuwa-Peters OL, Okafor SI, et al. Differential outcomes among survivors of head and neck cancer belonging to racial and ethnic minority groups. JAMA Otolaryngol Head & Neck Surgery 2022;148(2):119–27.
26. Pagedar NA, Davis AB, Sperry SM, et al. Population analysis of socioeconomic status and otolaryngologist distribution on head and neck cancer outcomes. Head Neck 2019;41(4):1046–52.
27. Naghavi AO, Echevarria MI, Grass GD, et al. Having Medicaid insurance negatively impacts outcomes in patients with head and neck malignancies. Cancer 2016;122(22):3529–37.
28. Inverso G, Mahal BA, Aizer AA, et al. Health insurance affects head and neck cancer treatment patterns and outcomes. J Oral Maxillofac Surg 2016/06/2016; 74(6):1241–7.
29. Kana LA, Graboyes EM, Quan D, et al. Association of changes in medicaid dental benefits with localized diagnosis of oral cavity cancer. JAMA Oncol 2022;8(5): 778–80.
30. Sineshaw HM, Ellis MA, Yabroff KR, et al. Association of medicaid expansion under the affordable care act with stage at diagnosis and time to treatment initiation for patients with head and neck squamous cell carcinoma. JAMA Otolaryngol Head Neck Surg 2020;146(3):247–55.
31. Frosch ZAK. Where have we been with rural-urban cancer care disparities and where are we headed? JAMA Netw Open 2022;5(5):e2212255.
32. Lawrence LA, Heuermann ML, Javadi P, et al. Socioeconomic status and rurality among patients with head and neck cancer. Otolaryngology-Head Neck Surg (Tokyo) 2022;166(6):1028–37.
33. Graboyes EM, Kompelli AR, Neskey DM, et al. Association of treatment delays with survival for patients with head and neck cancer: a systematic review. JAMA Otolaryngology–Head & Neck Surgery 2019;145(2):166–77.
34. Murphy CT, Galloway TJ, Handorf EA, et al. Survival impact of increasing time to treatment initiation for patients with head and neck cancer in the United States. J Clin Oncol 2016;34(2):169–78.
35. Foley J, Wishart LR, Ward EC, et al. Exploring the impact of remoteness on people with head and neck cancer: Utilisation of a state-wide dataset. Aust J Rural Health 2023;31(4):726–43.
36. Graboyes EM, Garrett-Mayer E, Sharma AK, et al. Adherence to National Comprehensive Cancer Network guidelines for time to initiation of postoperative radiation therapy for patients with head and neck cancer. Cancer 2017;123(14): 2651–60.
37. Guttmann DM, Kobie J, Grover S, et al. National disparities in treatment package time for resected locally advanced head and neck cancer and impact on overall survival. Head Neck 2018;40(6):1147–55.
38. National Comprehensive Cancer Network (NCCN). NCCN clinical practice guidelines in oncology (NCCN guidelines): head and neck cancers, National Comprehensive Cancer Network 2023. Plymouth Meeting, PA.
39. Graboyes EM, Divi V, Moore BA. Head and Neck Oncology Is on the National Quality Sidelines No Longer-Put Me in, Coach. JAMA otolaryngology– head & neck surgery 2022;148(8):715–6.

40. Lewis CM, Ajmani GS, Kyrillos A, et al. Racial disparities in the choice of definitive treatment for squamous cell carcinoma of the oral cavity. Head Neck 2018; 40(11):2372–82.

41. Nocon CC, Ajmani GS, Bhayani MK. A contemporary analysis of racial disparities in recommended and received treatment for head and neck cancer. Cancer 2020;126(2):381–9.

42. Benchetrit L, Torabi SJ, Tate JP, et al. Gender disparities in head and neck cancer chemotherapy clinical trials participation and treatment. Oral Oncol 2019;94: 32–40.

43. Russo DP, Tham T, Bardash Y, et al. The effect of race in head and neck cancer: A meta-analysis controlling for socioeconomic status. Am J Otolaryngol 2020/11/2020;41(6):102624.

44. Liu JC, Egleston BL, Blackman E, et al. Racial survival disparities in head and neck cancer clinical trials. J Natl Cancer Inst 2023;115(3):288–94.

45. Parasher AK, Abramowitz M, Weed D, et al. Ethnicity and clinical outcomes in head and neck cancer: an analysis of the SEER Database. Journal of Racial and Ethnic Health Disparities 2014;1(4):267–74.

46. Choi SH, Terrell JE, Fowler KE, et al. Socioeconomic and other demographic disparities predicting survival among head and neck cancer patients. PLoS One 2016;11(3):e0149886.

47. Lenze NR, Farquhar D, Sheth S, et al. Socioeconomic Status Drives Racial Disparities in HPV-negative Head and Neck Cancer Outcomes. Laryngoscope 2021;131(6):1301–9.

48. Pannu JS, Simpson MC, Adjei Boakye E, et al. Survival outcomes for head and neck patients with Medicaid: A health insurance paradox. Head Neck 2021; 43(7):2136–47.

49. Olsen MH, Bøje CR, Kjær TK, et al. Socioeconomic position and stage at diagnosis of head and neck cancer - a nationwide study from DAHANCA. Acta Oncol 2015;54(5):759–66.

50. Noyes EA, Burks CA, Larson AR, et al. An equity-based narrative review of barriers to timely postoperative radiation therapy for patients with head and neck squamous cell carcinoma. Laryngoscope Investig Otolaryngol 2021;6(6): 1358–66.

51. Guerriero MK, Redman MW, Baker KK, et al. Racial disparity in oncologic and quality-of-life outcomes in patients with locally advanced head and neck squamous cell carcinomas enrolled in a randomized phase 2 trial. Cancer 2018; 124(13):2841–9.

52. Adamowicz JL, Christensen A, Howren MB, et al. Health-related quality of life in head and neck cancer survivors: Evaluating the rural disadvantage. J Rural Health 2022;38(1):54–62.

53. Rieke K, Boilesen E, Lydiatt W, et al. Population-based retrospective study to investigate preexisting and new depression diagnosis among head and neck cancer patients. Cancer Epidemiol 2016;43:42–8.

54. Acuña-Villaorduña A, Baranda JC, Boehmer J, et al. Equitable access to clinical trials: how do we achieve it? Am Soc Clin Oncol Educ Book 2023;(43):e389838.

55. Scharff DP, Mathews KJ, Jackson P, et al. More than Tuskegee: understanding mistrust about research participation. J Health Care Poor Underserved 2010; 21(3):879–97.

56. Loree JM, Anand S, Dasari A, et al. Disparity of race reporting and representation in clinical trials leading to cancer drug approvals From 2008 to 2018. JAMA Oncol 2019;5(10):e191870.

57. Corbie-Smith G, Thomas SB, St. George DMM. Distrust, race, and research. Arch Intern Med 2002;162(21):2458–63.
58. Sauer AB, Daher GS, Lohse CM, et al. Underreporting and underrepresentation of race and ethnicity in head and neck cancer trials, 2010-2020: a systematic review. JAMA Otolaryngology–Head & Neck Surgery 2022;148(7):662–9.
59. U.S Food and Drug Administration. Diversity plans to improve enrollment of participants from underrepresented racial and ethnic populations in clinical trials. 2022. Available at: https://www.fda.gov/regulatory-information/search-fda-guidance-documents/diversity-plans-improve-enrollment-participants-underrepresented-racial-and-ethnic-populations.
60. Dymanus KA, Butaney M, Magee DE, et al. Assessment of gender representation in clinical trials leading to FDA approval for oncology therapeutics between 2014 and 2019: A systematic review-based cohort study. Cancer 2021;127(17): 3156–62.
61. Entezami P, Thomas B, Mansour J, et al. Targets for improving disparate head and neck cancer outcomes in the low-income population. Laryngoscope Investig Otolaryngol 2021;6(6):1481–8.
62. Jiang C, Yabroff KR, Deng L, et al. Self-reported transportation barriers to health care among US cancer survivors. JAMA Oncol 2022;8(5):775–8.
63. Salinas M, Chintakuntlawar A, Arasomwan I, et al. Emerging disparities in prevention and survival outcomes for patients with head and neck cancer and recommendations for health equity. Curr Oncol Rep 2022;24(9):1153–61.
64. Graboyes EM, Sterba KR, Li H, et al. Development and evaluation of a navigation-based, multilevel intervention to improve the delivery of timely, guideline-adherent adjuvant therapy for patients with head and neck cancer. JCO Oncol Pract 2021; 17(10):e1512–23.
65. Graboyes EM, Hill EG, Sterba KR, et al. Efficacy of a navigation-based intervention vs usual care for decreasing delays in starting guideline- adherent adjuvant therapy for patients with head and neck cancer. Philadelphia, PA. Abstract: IJROBP; 2024.
66. Graboyes EM, Chaiyachati KH, Sisto Gall J, et al. Addressing transportation insecurity among patients with cancer. J Natl Cancer Inst 2022;114(12):1593–600.
67. Eckhert E, Lansinger O, Ritter V, et al. Breast cancer diagnosis, treatment, and outcomes of patients from sex and gender minority groups. JAMA Oncol 2023; 9(4):473–80.
68. Ramakodi MP, Devarajan K, Blackman E, et al. Integrative genomic analysis identifies ancestry-related expression quantitative trait loci on DNA polymerase β and supports the association of genetic ancestry with survival disparities in head and neck squamous cell carcinoma. Cancer 2017;123(5):849–60.

Ethics and Palliation in Head and Neck Surgery

Colleen G. Hochfelder, MD, MS, Andrew G. Shuman, MD*

KEYWORDS

- Head and neck cancer • Medical ethics • Palliation • Shared decision-making

KEY POINTS

- Ethical dilemmas arising among patients with head and neck cancer are amplified by their vulnerability given challenges involving communication barriers and socioeconomic disparities.
- Shared decision-making for complicated choices in head and neck surgical oncology is improved with the application of tailored decision support tools and strategies.
- Upstream integration of palliative care and proactive efforts to address symptom burden and distress are critical for many patients with head and neck cancer even when cancer-directed therapy continues.

INTRODUCTION

Patients with head and neck cancer face a potentially traumatizing disease. These cancers can erode a patient's ability to perform many of the most basic human functions: eating, drinking, breathing, and speaking. Both the disease as well as treatment can cause temporary or permanent changes to patients' appearance, function, and ability to communicate, any of which can erode a patient's self-image, regardless of whether others would detect the same deficits.[1,2]

The management of such a challenging disease is made more complicated by the stigma associated with it. Tobacco and alcohol use/dependence have long been known risk factors for head and neck cancer, and patients with these "vice-related" cancers suffer stigma and shame.[3,4] Additional complexities arise from association with high-risk human papillomavirus (HPV) strains. Diagnosis with an HPV-related cancer can negatively affect patients who experience the embarrassment and shame of a sexually transmitted infection.[5] Low socioeconomic status, including low income and low education levels, is another independent risk factor for head and neck cancer.[6]

Many patients diagnosed with advanced stage disease, particularly those that are not HPV associated, will ultimately suffer recurrence and/or cancer-related mortality.[7]

Department of Otolaryngology–Head and Neck Surgery, University of Michigan, 1500 East Medical Center Drive, 1903 Taubman Center, SPC 5312, Ann Arbor, MI 48109-5312, USA
* Corresponding author.
E-mail address: shumana@med.umich.edu

Surg Oncol Clin N Am 33 (2024) 683–695
https://doi.org/10.1016/j.soc.2024.04.005
surgonc.theclinics.com

Over the past decade, survival for recurrent/metastatic disease has almost doubled (at least partially explained by the rise in HPV-related disease), but overall remains poor with median survival of less than a year after diagnosis.[8] With dismal outcomes among at least a sizable subset of patients, a focus upon palliation is of vital importance for patients with head and neck cancer.

Diagnosis with head and neck cancer leaves patients who are already disadvantaged in a uniquely vulnerable position when interacting with the medical system.[9] Decision-making is especially fraught when ethical dilemmas arise in this population.[10] Herein, the authors will review foundational ethical principles and frameworks to guide care of these patients. The authors will further discuss specific ethical conflicts relevant for patients with head and neck cancer including shared decision-making (SDM) and advance care planning. The authors will discuss palliative care with a discussion of the role of surgery as a component of palliation at multiple stages of the disease trajectory.

Medical Ethics in Head and Neck Cancer

Clinical ethics involves the moral deliberation involved with balancing clinical obligations with the needs, preferences, and rights of patients and society.[11–14] Special considerations nuance the unique relationships and power dynamics within the medical field. A distinct field of medical ethics is research ethics. In clinical research, subjects opt to participate in investigations designed for the good of scientific advancement while accepting an augmented risk of harm.[11,15] While research ethics are of utmost concern and relevance for those engaged in head and neck oncology preclinical and clinical trials, the authors will mainly focus on clinical ethics herein.

Ethical theories and frameworks have developed and been adapted to offer systematic approaches to address dilemmas arising in clinical care. A straightforward approach for providers to use is the application of widely accepted ethical values which together can be used to describe and address myriad issues that arise in clinical practice. The 4 guiding principles—autonomy, beneficence, non-maleficence, and justice—together comprise a framework and working language for the field.[16–18] Autonomy is the right of the patient to determine and decide what interventions may take place in their own body.[11,16,17] The underlying assumption is that ultimately patients have the authority to make decisions about their own life, especially if the results of a decision only affect a single individual. Beneficence dictates that clinicians should act in the best interest of their patient.[11,16] Non-maleficence encompasses the requirement for providers to avoid and/or mitigate harm to their patients.[11,16] Justice was one of Aristotle's 4 cardinal virtues; John Rawls considered justice "the first virtue of social institutions."[19] This belies the concept that patients should be treated with the same high-quality evidence-based care regardless of age, culture, religion, class, or any other individual trait. While there are many other approaches and frameworks within clinical ethics, principlism is a relatively straightforward and well-established approach that can be complementary and is an approachable methodology for those without formal training in ethics.[16–18]

Shared Decision-Making in Head and Neck Oncology

SDM is a widely accepted model for providing clinical care. This can often introduce ethical conflicts as both the patient and the provider act as moral agents in this model.[20] SDM requires a collaboration between patients and providers leveraging the clinical knowledge and expertise of the provider to make decisions in line with the preferences and values of the patient.[21] Application of SDM varies widely; there are differing perspectives on how much information should be shared by both parties, what degree of patient involvement is optimal or acceptable, and how to protect and guide patients who prefer to defer decisions to others.[21] Numerous models have been developed to build a framework for SDM. Makoul and Clayman[22] incorporated related values and themes and proposed an integrative model of SDM built from 9 key characteristics emphasized in the literature. These characteristics included the following: defining/explaining the problem, presenting treatment options, reviewing the pros and cons, consideration of the patient's values and preferences, consideration of the patient's ability and self-efficacy, considering the physician's knowledge and recommendations, clarifying the patient's understanding, deciding, or postponing decision, and ensuring follow-up.

Numerous other models have been described in oncology including methods of implementation at a systems level. Bomhof-Roordink described an SDM model developed from common themes taken from interviews of oncology patients, providers, and researchers.[23] Multiple clinical decision-making tools have also been developed to help guide clinicians. There have been calls for further development of quantitative, validated tools for eliciting patient preferences and values to guide SDM.[24] Still despite the growing literature around specific models and tools, more data are needed to guide implementation of specific, validated tools within head and neck surgery.[21] Consideration of patient-centered approaches are essential for development of clinical decision-making tools. For a subset of patients, they may prefer to defer decisions to their providers or defer decisions beyond the decision to treat or not to treat.[25]

There is concern that while SDM may be more readily integrated during curative-intent therapy, in the case of advanced and progressive disease, when options may be limited, this may break down. Qualitative studies of patients and physicians around therapeutic options for advanced cancer, including a subset of head and neck cancer patients, report that uncertainty about the risk-benefit ratio of therapies for patients led to breakdown in the ability to adhere to an SDM model.[26] Despite SDM being more challenging to employ toward the end of life, patients have a desire for more input and control over these deliberations, from life-and-death decisions to more mundane ones. A review of the palliative and hospice nursing literature finds that patients are more satisfied with an SDM approach across these spectrums.[27]

Informed consent is an essential component to providing contemporary medical care. Consent hinges on the exchange of information from the provider to the patient or their surrogate decision maker with the positive affirmation of desire for the intervention being offered.[28] The American Medical Association (AMA) has provided clear guidance on what criteria are needed to achieve informed consent. Physicians are required to assess the patient's or surrogate decision maker's ability to understand medical information and implications of a decision for a given treatment or its alternatives. The physician must provide relevant information about the diagnosis; the nature and purpose of interventions; and the burdens, risks, benefits of all options, including no treatment. The physician has an ensuing obligation to document these discussions and the patient's preferences/ultimate choices.[29]

One of the difficulties of oncologic care is ensuring that patients have adequate understanding of their disease, the treatment options, and possible negative effects of various treatments including foregoing cancer-directed therapy.[30] For patients considering surgical intervention, undue emphasis may be placed on compliance aspects of ensuring documentation rather than truly ensuring that patients and families are duly informed. Most physicians receive little to no formal training in providing informed consent.[31,32] Surveys of surgical interns have found that less than 40% report having formal training in obtaining informed consent, and most report that their education around consent involved watching other trainees and replicating their process.[33]

Reliance on written documents to provide information may also be insufficient. An analysis of surgical consent forms using the Flesch-Kincaid formula to calculate reading level found that forms in the United Kingdom, Germany, Austria, and Switzerland all required at least a high-school level education and most required post-secondary education to comprehend.[34] A study of guidelines from the American, British, and Canadian otolaryngology—head and neck surgery societies demonstrated they are similarly published at a high-school reading level. The head and neck oncology guidelines across these societies were published at a ninth grade level.[35]

These issues are particularly germane in head and neck cancer. A review of 31 studies from 27 countries found that 38% of head and neck cancer patients had an educational level equivalent to elementary/middle school and 35% had the equivalent of secondary education.[6] This suggests that only a quarter of head and neck cancer patients would be able to read and comprehend either guidelines or a surgical consent form. Written documents for complex surgery and reconstruction could be expected to be largely indecipherable for the average patient. Instead of solely relying on written documents, there is a role for advanced decision-making tools with patients such as decision aids and/or video/multimedia formats.

The development of decision-making tools specific for head and neck cancer is ongoing. This is best achieved using mixed methods and multiple routes of inquiry to evaluate quantitative metrics as well as qualitative ones, such as values and beliefs. Forner and colleagues[36] proposed the need for specific SDM tools for the care of advanced oral cavity cancer. To initiate the development of such a tool, Forner and colleagues[36] proposed a stakeholder needs evaluation using mixed-methods including validated-quantitative measures of degree of SDM, patient confidence, and decisional conflict, as well as semi-structured interviews to evaluate values and beliefs. Meticulous development of SDM tools specific to head and neck cancer could be applied to further clinical scenarios within head and neck to improve ability to achieve SDM. An ongoing challenge of these tools is the need to update them as data and practice guidelines evolve.

Patients with head and neck cancer often suffer from unique communication challenges which may make more classical medical interviewing more difficult. Pretreatment speech deficits have been reported as affecting 46% of patients, especially those with laryngeal cancer.[37] Whenever feasible, clinicians should also spend more time explaining the procedure and risks with the patient to improve the degree of understanding and use augmented approaches to mitigate inherent barriers.[28]

Communication breakdowns are a frequent component leading to ethical dilemmas in clinical practice. Shuman and colleagues[38] conducted a study of ethical consultations at 2 large academic institutes and found that the most common conflicts were surrounding code status and advance directives (25%), surrogate decision making (17%), and concerns about medical futility. Underlying problems with poor communication were identified in 45% of cases with resulting conflict between providers and families or a combination of the 2.[38,39]

One validated method called "best case/worst case" offers a means for surgeons to communicate clearly about surgical choices.[40] This tool involves the surgeon drawing a linear spectrum of expected outcomes with surgery and without surgery. The surgeon walks the patient through the options from best case to worst case with each option. This tool was developed through focus groups with both surgeons and elderly adults who lauded the ability to use the tool to elicit a patient's goals and understand the limitations of surgery. The tool was subsequently taught to surgeons.[41] Surgeons who underwent formal teaching of use of the "best case/worst case" tool had significantly improved scores in third-party observer scoring of degree of SDM.[41] This tool does have limitations. The opinions about what is the best case/worst case are somewhat subjective and inherently influenced by the surgeon's biases.[40]

Operative Decision-Making

Operative consent represents a unique subset of the informed consent process within medicine. The operating room poses a distinct environment as the patient is in the most vulnerable of settings. Surgical consent is a form of batched consent in which patients agree to undergo surgery, but in so doing are agreeing all the standard perioperative care that a surgery entails. Unique challenges within surgery include unexpected findings and immediate management of those problems. Langerman[42] describes informed consent as incorporating an "advance surgical directive." In an ideal situation, the surgical team would have discussed all likely possibilities prior to the surgery and would have a detailed and nuanced understanding of a patient's wishes prior to anesthesia. But for many unexpected surgical events, this is not feasible. In this case, a surrogate decision maker may offer the chance for the patient's wishes to be known and respected until they regain capacity to make their own decisions.

It is worth noting that studies of surrogate decision makers in end-of-life care have found discordance between the decisions made by the surrogate and those that the patient would make for themselves. Shalowitz[43] performed a systematic review and found only a 68% concordance between surrogate decisions and patient preferences. Ultimately, the surgeon must adhere to the principles of beneficence and nonmaleficence in their intraoperative care. Where delay would incur unreasonable risk to the patient, the surgeon should act in the patient's best interest, absent other clear knowledge of their preferences.[42] The AMA's ethical guidelines on informed consent address emergencies and unexpected contingencies. The AMA requires that in the case that the patient or surrogate decision maker is not available, the physician should act in the best interest of the patient and as soon as the patient or surrogate is available, they must obtain consent for ongoing care.[29]

Another caveat to surgical decision-making is the concept of surgical "buy-in." Surgeons frequently view the preoperative consenting process as a mutual contract in which a patient agrees to a window of recovery following a surgery. Surgeons are reluctant to limit interventions or deviate from standard practice in this perioperative window, and experience distress if a patient wants to alter the treatment plan or decline aspects of care even in the face of complications and turbulent clinical trajectories.[43] Surgeons gain buy-in and communicate information about the risks and possible negative outcomes for surgery by emphasizing that the patient is facing a "big surgery," but few explicitly discussed the use of prolonged life support or other aggressive interventions.[44] Surgeons encourage questions, but much of their conversation with the patient may revolve around technical aspects of surgery and subsequent care. They do not necessarily discuss larger questions about values, goals, and discussion of management in worst-case scenarios.[45] This highlights the potential role of "best case/worst case."[41]

Communicating the risks and potential outcomes for major interventions can be challenging and lead to difficult conversations. In scenarios where surgeons discuss patient preferences and patients express a desire for an advance directive limiting postoperative life-supporting therapy, some surgeons would hesitate to operate.[46] Indeed, surgeons have conflicted views of advance directives in perioperative care.[47] In qualitative studies, surgeons' express frustrations about the gaps between written advance directives and the realities of complex medical decision-making.[47] But the encouragement of detailed advance directives allows a patient's wishes to be understood and is of paramount importance, particularly for high-risk procedures such as major head and neck surgeries.[48]

The American College of Surgeons issued a statement in 2014 on the required reconsideration of code status prior to surgery with discussion of intraoperative and perioperative risks and how those fit with the patient's treatment goals.[49] Further, they recommended discussion and planning for care in the event of potentially life-threatening problems including patients/families, surgeons, perioperative nurses, and the anesthesia team.[49] Integration of palliative care specialists into the surgical oncologic care in parallel to cancer-directed treatment has been associated with higher rates of advance directive documentation and better synergy in alignment of goals.[50]

Critical to management in surgical oncology are decisions about resectability. Resectability is perhaps more subjective than one might assume. The decision about if a tumor is resectable includes considerations about anatomic bounds of a tumor and expected margins, but also includes considerations about a patient's medical fitness, oncologic prognosis, genetic/molecular features of the tumor, and anticipated post-operative function.[51] The surgeon's gestalt of a patient may shape decisions about medical fitness for surgery and is highly susceptible to bias, inconsistency, and lack of interrater reliability.[52] Careful and deliberate multidisciplinary reflection on the criteria for determining resectability and subsequently making the decision of whether to offer an operation must be a standard practice for the head and neck surgeon.

Palliative Care in Head and Neck Cancer

Many patients with head and neck cancer are diagnosed with advanced stage disease, and many will ultimately develop locoregional recurrence or distant metastasis resulting in significant morbidity and risk of cancer-related mortality.[7] Progressive and incurable head and neck cancer particularly with uncontrolled locoregional disease is a horrible condition. Patients face refractory pain; the inability to eat, drink, or speak; anorexia and cachexia; delirium; inability to manage their secretions; airway obstruction and air hunger; tumor bleeding; fistulae; and nonhealing wounds.[53]

Supportive care has an important role to play. Humidification and oral care can prevent tumors from crusting, ulcerating, and bleeding. Wound care and local hygiene can help to control odor and reduce bacterial burden. Multimodal and multidisciplinary medical management has a huge role to play with the use of analgesics, suppression of secretions, topical antibiotics for malodorous tumors, and systemic antibiotics for recurrent infections of fistulae.[53] Steroids can drive appetite and address edema at least temporarily.

Many of these symptoms in patients with incurable disease can be managed in part with palliative chemotherapy and/or brief courses of palliative radiation. Some of the complications are more challenging to manage with medications alone. Tumor bleeding or rupture of major branches of the external carotid artery as the tumor invades these arteries can be dramatic and life threatening. This can pose significant morbidity and mortality to patients, and devastating trauma to caregivers who watch their loved ones suffer massive hemorrhage.[53] If feasible, intervention by neuroradiology may be an option as a component of palliation. In the terminally ill patient with nonresectable disease, education, counseling, and clear communication about the patient's wishes in such an instance are essential. Airway obstruction similarly can be mitigated by tracheostomy even if that will not change the underlying pathology or prognosis.[53] Patients benefit greatly from multidisciplinary expertise, especially the inclusion of palliative care physicians.[38,54]

Traditional models of care may involve abrupt transition from curative-intent care to palliative symptom management with palliation pursued once curative or cancer-directed therapy is no longer feasible. Patients and surgeons carry cultural biases and an approach to cancer which can influence their decisions about whether to operate. When President Nixon declared "war on cancer" in 1971, the collective consciousness reframed cancer care using this metaphor involving a fight until death.[55] Cancer care in the following decades has evolved and many cancers have changed from a death sentence to a chronic disease.[55] In the context of chronic care or in the palliative setting, the war metaphor can be problematic as it encourages "fighting" at all costs. There are efforts to change the narrative around cancer care to focus on "leaving no patient behind" and emphasizing quality of life rather than "soldiering on."[55,56] This old-fashioned view of care may lead to a failure to incorporate proactive attention to and management of symptoms.

The American Society of Clinical Oncology recommends the integration of palliative care early in care of patients with advanced cancers.[57] A concurrent approach, where patients receive curative-intent care and palliative care, offers improvement for quality of life, survival, and patient satisfaction.[58] Curative and palliative therapies should be seen as partners rather than mutually exclusive approaches. Surgery for a head and neck cancer may offer a chance at improved survival but can also offer reduction in pain, and restoration of function. Surgery for advanced head and neck cancer can be viewed in this regard as both curative and palliative in intent.[58,59]

There is a growing role for surgery with palliative intent among patients with cancer. Highly selected patients may benefit from operations intended to reduce cancer pain, improve the degree of disfigurement, and decrease suffering from fistulae or large wounds.[58–61] The burden of shared decision is even greater in palliative scenarios where the outcomes may be harder to predict, and the stakes may be fundamentally different. In the palliative setting, surgeons must be extra diligent in counseling their patients and ensure the proposed surgery fits certain essential criteria. The surgeon must ensure that the procedure is consistent with the patient's wishes and goals of care, with reasonably achievable goals. The surgeon must ensure that the patient has realistic expectations and consider the balance of potential risks and potential benefits. Finally, in the palliative setting, the patient must have a life expectancy long enough to recover from surgery and enjoy the potential benefits.

Surgical palliative care is emerging as a new field.[62,63] Within that umbrella, surgeons with specialized training in both head and neck oncology and palliative care can drive this field forward and improve care for head and neck cancer patients. Early career surgeons with an interest in palliative care should consider additional specialized training and education.[63]

Emerging Ethical Issues in Head and Neck Cancer

There are many emerging ethical issues relevant to the field of head and neck surgical oncology. The role of physician-assisted suicide (PAS) has undergone significant debate among philosophers, clinicians, lawyers, ethicists, and policymakers. The unique physical and psychological toll on patients with advanced and incurable head and neck cancer may make this of growing relevance in the future. Currently, a minority of states have laws allowing for PAS.[64] There is a relative dearth of data informing this issue among head and neck cancer patients. Kligerman and Divi[65] reviewed records from Oregon where PAS is legal under their Death with Dignity Act. Over a 20-year period, 57 patients with advanced terminal head and neck cancer were enrolled and provided prescriptions for medications to end their lives. Of these, 39 ended their lives with these drugs. Those who used the medications were significantly less educated compared to their counterparts who received the medications but opted not to use them.[65] This represents only a small cohort of patients with advanced head and neck cancer, and of those who received a prescription, only a subset used the medication. Studies of physician opinion on PAS have found that a slight majority (57%) of physicians feel the practice should be legal and roughly half report that they would ever personally consider providing lethal doses of medications to a patient.[64] This is an understandably controversial issue, and the ethical and legal context of PAS will continue to evolve.

Another area of conflicting values involves the implementation of telehealth. Telehealth poses potential issues with care fragmentation. Patients receiving care via telehealth through multiple care systems and providers might be at risk of poorer communication between people and teams. This may exacerbate transitions of care and communication between key members of the interdisciplinary team, for example, between medical and radiation oncologists in a patient's hometown and a patient's head and neck surgeon at a tertiary care center. Care fragmentation is already a major issue in care of cancer patients. Aiello Bowles and colleagues[30] surveyed experts through the National Cancer Institute. A major criticism of oncologic care was poor multidisciplinary teamwork with communication breakdowns leading to delays in care especially at periods of transition of care. Additionally, the reliance on telehealth may erode the doctor-patient relationship. While video visits are becoming more common, satisfaction can vary among patient populations. Some early survey data have shown patients with head and neck cancer appreciate the convenience of a video visit.[66,67] Still, other surveys of patient experience have mixed results. A survey of telehealth services through the Department of Veterans Affairs found that about one-third of the patients had positive experiences, while one-third reported neutral experiences, and the remianing one-third reported negative experiences.[68] The promise of telehealth offers a route to increased health care equity and more fair distribution of care. Telehealth could be used to increase the access of rural, disabled, and impoverished patients, but the gaps in access to high-speed internet poses systemic hurdles for many patients.[69,70] As recently as the end of 2017, 26% of rural Americans and 32% of Native Americans on tribal land lacked access to high-speed Internet.[70] With increasing complexity and cost of health care coupled with an ever-evolving marker of payers and providers, telehealth will pose an ongoing challenge as well as opportunity.

The role of precision medicine also poses new ethical considerations. Genomic characterization of cancer is allowing for personalized tailored therapies.[71,72] Precision medicine in this way blurs the distinction between clinical care and research.[73] Clinical trials may offer the opportunity to evaluate tumor biology and attempt to target these mutations with novel biologic therapies. The goal of such research is to increase generalizable knowledge rather than therapeutic benefit for an individual.[15,74] But patient's expectations about personal benefit are harder to manage. Physicians may also harbor high optimism about interventions offered in a trial may benefit their patient and be more likely to provide directive counseling.[61] In addition, precision oncology may be incorporated into clinical practice despite a relative dearth of conclusive research into its potential value in specific circumstances. Bias is another concern particularly given that data-informing approaches and protocols may have been devised from homogenous patient populations. Implementation of precision medicine requires implementation with the utmost dedication to preventing distorted use of genetic information to reenforce systematic biases about disadvantaged groups. Further, it requires delivery in a manner to address social determinants of health rather than re-enforce inequities.[75]

Health care resource allocation remains a perennial concern. Global allocation of resources continues to represent a major ethical issue with large inequities globally. In 2016, the Lancet Commission on Global Surgery led an international conference to gain buy-in from high-income country (HIC) clinicians and politicians and to develop an international consensus approach to improving global access to surgery.[76] The commission set several recommendations including creating responsibility for HIC organizations for inequities, moving away from surgical colonialism, supporting academic research in low-income and middle-income countries (LMIC), and investments by global health leaders and industry in LMIC.[76]

Delivery of timely surgical care for head and neck cancer patients was derailed globally by the coronavirus disease 2019 pandemic with potential consequences on disease control and patient outcomes. Considering limited resources, the Surgical Prioritization and Ranking Tool and Navigation Aid for Head and Neck Cancer, a surgical prioritization algorithm, was developed by expert consensus using a modified Delphi process.[77] Designed for the initial pandemic, the use of such a prioritization algorithm provides tools for navigating a continued burdened health care system with limited resources. In many ways, the pandemic highlighted issues of inequity within and across borders and the specific hurdles challenges in delivering equitable care for head and neck cancer patients. This applies to macro-level decisions regarding where surgical care is offered, down to micro-level decisions as individual surgeons triage patients for their finite operative block time.

SUMMARY

Ethically informed and appropriate care of individuals with head and neck cancer requires thoughtfulness, honesty, and fortitude. Underlying normative ethical theories and approaches offer broad guidance that must then be applied with disease-specific and specialty-specific expertise. Areas of focus for patients with head and neck cancer include the role of SDM and informed consent, and the role of palliative surgery. Ultimately, the crux of high-quality ethical care of patients with head and neck cancer centers on ensuring there is excellent communication between the provider and the patient to allow for honest dissemination of patient-centric information, in-depth exploration of a patient's values and goals, and alignment of therapeutic options with the patient's desires.

CLINICS CARE POINTS

- Head and neck cancer patients are uniquely vunerable to ethical dilemmas. These dilemmas most commonly arise around decision-making and end of life care. Use of a shared-decision making toold and a multi-disciplinary team approach offer means to mitigate these conflicts.

- The key to achieving high-quality ethical care of head and neck cancer patints is investing in excellent communication between providers and patients with education on the disease process, in-depth exploration of the patient's values and goals, and alignment of the therapeutic options to fit within the patient's desires.

DISCLOSURE

The authors have nothing to disclose.

REFERENCES

1. Macias D, Hand BN, Zenga J, et al. Association Between Observer-Rated Disfigurement and Body Image-Related Distress Among Head and Neck Cancer Survivors. JAMA Otolaryngol Head Neck Surg 2022;148(7):688–9.
2. Henry M, Albert JG, Frenkiel S, et al. Body Image Concerns in Patients With Head and Neck Cancer: A Longitudinal Study. Front Psychol 2022;13:816587.
3. Blot WJ, McLaughlin JK, Winn DM, et al. Smoking and drinking in relation to oral and pharyngeal cancer. Cancer Res 1988;48:3282–7.
4. Warner ET, Park ER, Luberto CM, et al. Internalized stigma among cancer patients enrolled in a smoking cessation trial: The role of cancer type and associations with psychological distress. Psycho Oncol 2022;31(5):753–60.
5. Dodd RH, Forster AS, Marlow LAV, et al. Psychosocial impact of human papillomavirus-related head and neck cancer on patients and their partners: A qualitative interview study. Eur J Cancer Care 2019;28(2):e12999.
6. Conway DI, Brenner DR, McMahon AD, et al. Estimating and explaining the effect of education and income on head and neck cancer risk: INHANCE consortium pooled analysis of 31 case-control studies from 27 countries. Int J Cancer 2015;136(5):1125–39.
7. Argiris A, Karamouzis MV, Raben D, et al. Head and neck cancer. Lancet 2008; 371:1695–709.
8. Haring CT, Kana LA, Dermody SM, et al. Patterns of recurrence in head and neck squamous cell carcinoma to inform personalized surveillance protocols. Cancer 2023;129(18):2817–27.
9. Schneck DP. Ethical considerations in the treatment of head and neck cancer. Cancer Control 2002;9(5):410–9.
10. Conley J. Ethics in Otolaryngology. Acta Otolaryngol 1981;91(1–6):369–74.
11. Taylor RM. Ethical principles and concepts in medicine. Handb Clin Neurol 2013; 118:1–9.
12. Jonsen AR, Siegler M, Winslade WJ. Clinical ethics: a practical approach to ethical decisions in clinical medicine. 9th edition. New York, NY: McGraw-Hill; 2022.
13. Lo B, Malina D, Pittman G, et al. Fundamentals of medical ethics – a new perspective series. N Engl J Med 2023;389(25):2392–4.
14. Lo B. Resolving ethical dilemmas: a guide for clinicians. 4th edition. Philadelphia, PA: Wolters Kluwer Health/Lippincott Williams & Wilkins; 2009.
15. Smith JD, Birkeland AC, Goldman EB, et al. Immortal Life of the Common Rule: Ethics, Consent, and the Future of Cancer Research. J Clin Oncol 2017;35(17): 1879–83.
16. Beauchamp T, Childress J. Principles of biomedical ethics. 7th edition. New York: Oxford University Press; 2013.
17. Gillon R. Medical ethics: four principles plus attention to scope. BMJ 1994;309: 184–8.
18. Gillon R. Ethics needs principles—four can encompass the rest—and respect for autonomy should be "first among equals.". J Med Ethics 2003;29:307–12.
19. Miller D. "Justice", the stanford encyclopedia of philosophy (fall 2023 edition). Zalta E.N., Nodelman U., editors, Available at: https://plato.stanford.edu/archives/fall2023/entries/justice/. Accessed January 17, 2024.
20. Peppercorn J. Ethics of ongoing cancer care for patients making risky decisions. J Oncol Pract 2012;8(5):e111–3.

21. Forner D, Noel CW, Shuman AG, et al. Shared decision-making in head and neck surgery: a review. JAMA Otolaryngol Head Neck Surg 2020;146(9):839–44.
22. Makoul G, Clayman ML. An integrative model of shared decision making in medical encounters. Patient Educ Couns 2006;60(3):301–12.
23. Bomhof-Roordink H, Fischer MJ, Duijn-Bakker N, et al. Shared decision making in oncology: A model based on patients', health care professionals', and researchers' views. Psycho Oncol 2019;28(1):139–46.
24. Richardson DR, Loh KP. Improving personalized treatment decision-making for older adults with cancer: The necessity of eliciting patient preferences. J Geriatr Oncol 2022;13(1):1–3.
25. Davies L, Rhodes LA, Grossman DC, et al. Decision making in head and neck cancer care. Laryngoscope 2010;120(12):2434–45.
26. Beaussant Y, Mathieu-Nicot F, Pazart L, et al. Is shared decision-making vanishing at the end-of-life? A descriptive and qualitative study of advanced cancer patients' involvement in specific therapies decision-making. BMC Palliat Care 2015; 14:61.
27. Kuosmanen L, Hupli M, Ahtiluoto S, et al. Patient participation in shared decision-making in palliative care – an integrative review. J Clin Nurs 2021;30(23–24): 3415–28.
28. Grady C. Enduring and emerging challenges of informed consent. N Engl J Med 2015;372:855–62.
29. American Medical Association. 2.1.1 informed consent. AMA Code of Medical Ethics; 2016. Available at: www.ama-assn.org/delivering-care/ethics/code-medical-ethics-overview. [Accessed 28 January 2024].
30. Aiello Bowles EJ, Tuzzio L, Wiese CJ, et al. Understanding high-quality cancer care: a summary of expert perspectives. Cancer 2008;112(4):934–42.
31. Nickels AS, Tilburt JC, Ross LF. Pediatric Resident Preparedness and Educational Experiences With Informed Consent. Acad Pediatr 2016;16(3):298–304.
32. McClean KL, Card SE. Informed consent skills in internal medicine residency: how are residents taught, and what do they learn? Acad Med 2004;79(2):128–33.
33. Koller SE, Morre RF, Goldberg MB, et al. An informed consent program enhances surgery resident education. J Surg Educ 2017;74(5):906–13.
34. Lagler FB, Weinbeck SB, Schwab M. Enduring and emerging challenges of informed consent. N Engl J Med 2015;372(22):2170–1.
35. Kim JH, Grose E, Philteos J, et al. Readability of the American, Canadian, and British Otolaryngology-Head and Neck Surgery Societies' Patient Materials. Otolaryngol Head Neck Surg 2022;166(5):862–8.
36. Forner D, Hong P, Corsten M, et al. Needs assessment for a decision support tool in oral cancer requiring major resection and reconstruction: a mixed-methods study protocol. BMJ Open 2020;10(11):e036969.
37. Piai V, Jansen F, Dahlslätt K, et al. Prevalence of neurocognitive and perceived speech deficits in patients with head and neck cancer before treatment: Associations with demographic, behavioral, and disease-related factors. Head Neck 2022;44(2):332–44.
38. Shuman AG, Montas SM, Barnosky AR, et al. Clinical Ethics Consultation in Oncology. Journal of Oncology Practice 2013;9(5):240–5.
39. Shuman AG, McCabe MS, Fins JJ, et al. Clinical ethics consultation in patients with head and neck cancer. Head Neck 2013;35(11):1647–51.
40. Kruser JM, Nabozny MJ, Steffens NM, et al. "Best case/worst case": qualitative evaluation of a novel communication tool for difficult in-the-moment surgical decisions. J Am Geriatr Soc 2015;63(9):1805–11.

41. Taylor LJ, Nabozny MJ, Steffens NM, et al. A framework to improve surgeon communication in high-stakes surgical decisions: best case/worst case. JAMA Surg 2017;152(6):531–8.
42. Langerman A, Siegler M, Angelos P. Intraoperative Decision Making: The Decision to Perform Additional, Unplanned Procedures on Anesthetized Patients. J Am Coll Surg 2016;222(5):956–60.
43. Shalowitz DI, Garrett-Mayer E, Wendler D. The accuracy of surrogate decision makers: a systematic review. Arch Intern Med 2006;166:e439–97.
44. Pecanac KE, Kehler JM, Brasel KJ, et al. It's big surgery: preoperative expressions of risk, responsibility, and commitment to treatment after high-risk operations. Ann Surg 2014;259(3):458–63.
45. Schwartze ML, Bradley CT, Brasel KJ. Surgical "buy-in": The contractual relationship between surgeons and patients that influences decisions regarding life-supporting therapy. Crit Care Med 2010;38(3):843–8.
46. Redmann AJ, Brasel KJ, Alexander CG, et al. Use of advance directives for high-risk operations: a national survey of surgeons. Ann Surg 2012;255(3):418–23.
47. Bradley CT, Brasel KJ, Schwarze ML. Physician attitudes regarding advance directives for high-risk surgical patients: a qualitative analysis. Surgery 2010;148(2):209–16.
48. Cooper ZR, Powers CL, Cobb JP. Putting the patient first: honoring advance directives prior to surgery. Ann Surg 2012;255(3):424–6.
49. Board of Regents of the American College of Surgeons. Statement on advance directives by patients: "do not resuscitate" in the operating room. Bull Am Coll Surg 2014;99(1):42–3.
50. Bansal VV, Kim D, Reddy B, et al. Early integrated palliative care within a surgical oncology clinic. JAMA Netw Open 2023;6(11):e2341928.
51. Shuman AG. Contemplating resectability. Hastings Cent Rep 2017;47(6):3–4.
52. Binkley CE, Reynolds JM, Shuman AG. From the eyeball test to the algorithm – quality of life, disability status, and clinical decision making in surgery. N Engl J Med 2022;387(14):1325–8.
53. Shuman AG, Fins JJ, Prince MEP. Improving end-of-life care for head and neck cancer patients. Expet Rev Anticancer Ther 2012;12(3):35–343.
54. Hinshaw DB, Pawlik T, Mosenthal AC, et al. When do we stop, and how do we do it? Medical futility and withdrawal of care. J Am Coll Surg 2003;196(4):621–51.
55. Parikh RB, Kirch RA, Brawley OW. Advancing a quality-of-life agenda in cancer advocacy beyond the war metaphor. JAMA Oncol 2015;1(4):423–4.
56. Oronsky BT, Carter CA, Oronsky AL, et al. "No patient left behind": an alternative to "the War on Cancer" metaphor. Med Oncol 2016;33:55.
57. Ferrell BR, Temel JS, Temin S, et al. Integration of palliative care into standard oncology care: American Society of Clinical Oncology clinical practice guideline update. J Clin Oncol 2017;35(1):96–112.
58. Esce A, McCammon S. Holding curative and palliative intentions. AMA J Ethics 2021;23(10):E766–71.
59. McCammon SD. Concurrent palliative care in the surgical management of head and neck cancer. J Surg Oncol 2019;120:78–84.
60. Jorgensen J, Redman R, Jusufbegovic M. The ethics of palliative surgery for locally advanced head and neck squamous cell carcinoma. Otolaryngology-Head Neck Surg (Tokyo) 2023;169(3):738–40.
61. Ovaitt AK, McCammon S. Ethical considerations in caring for patients with advanced malignancy. Surg Oncol Clin N Am 2021;30(3):581–9.

62. McCammon SD, Hoffman MR. Development of surgical palliative care as a field and community building in palliative care: past, present, and future directions. Ann Palliat Med 2022;11(2):852–61.
63. Bassette E, Salyer C, McCammon S, et al. Hospice and palliative medicine fellowship after surgical training: a roadmap to the future of surgical palliative care. J Surg Educ 2022;79(5):1177–87.
64. Pai S, Andrews T, Turner A, et al. Factors that influence end-of-life decision making amongst attending physicians. Am J Hosp Palliat Care 2022;39(10):1174–81.
65. Kligerman MP, Divi V. Physician-assisted suicide for patients with head and neck cancer. Otolaryngology-Head Neck Surg (Tokyo) 2020;163(4):759–62.
66. Triantafillou V, Layfield E, Prasad A, et al. Patient perceptions of head and neck ambulatory telemedicine visits: a qualitative study. Otolaryngol Head Neck Surg 2021;164(5):923–31.
67. Dhillon K, Manji J, Céspedes MT, et al. Use of telemedicine consultations in head and neck cancer: patient perceptions, acceptability and accessibility. ANZ J Surg 2022;92(6):1415–22.
68. Slightam C, Gregory AJ, Hu J, et al. Patient perceptions of video visits using veterans affairs telehealth tablets: survey study. J Med Internet Res 2020;22(4):e15682.
69. Bauer K. Distributive justice and rural healthcare: a case for e-health. Int J Appl Philos 2003;17(2):241–52.
70. Sanders CK, Scanlon E. The digital divide is a human rights issue: advancing social inclusion through social work advocacy. J of Human Rights and Social Work 2021;6:130–43.
71. Chapman PB, Hauschild A, Robert C, et al. Improved survival with vemurafenib in melanoma with BRAF V600E mutation. N Engl J Med 2011;364:2507–16.
72. Slamon DJ, Leyland-Jones B, Shak S, et al. Use of chemotherapy plus a monoclonal antibody against HER2 for metastatic breast cancer that overex- presses HER2. N Engl J Med 2001;344:783–92.
73. Marchiano EJ, Birkeland AC, Swiecicki PL, et al. Revisiting expectations in an era of precision oncology. Oncol 2018;23(3):386–8.
74. Henderson GE, Churchill LR, Davis AM, et al. Clinical trials and medical care: defining the therapeutic misconception. PLoS Med 2007;4(11):e324.
75. Matthew DB. Two threats to precision medicine equity. Ethn Dis 2019;29(Suppl 3):629–40.
76. Ng-Kamstra JS, Greenberg SLM, Abdullah F, et al. Global surgery 2030: a roadmap for high income country actors. BMJ Glob Health 2016;1(1):e000011.
77. de Almeida JR, Noel CW, Forner D, et al. Development and validation of a surgical prioritization and ranking tool and navigation aid for head and neck cancer (SPARTAN-HN) in a scarce resource setting: response to the COVID-19 pandemic. Cancer 2020;126(22):4895–904.

Treatment De-escalation in Oropharyngeal Carcinoma and the Role of Robotic Surgery

John Ceremsak, MD*, Wenda Ye, MD, Melanie Hicks, MD, Kyle Mannion, MD

KEYWORDS

- Oropharynx • SCC • HPV • De-escalation • TORS

KEY POINTS

- Oropharyngeal squamous cell carcinoma (OPSCC) related to human papillomavirus (HPV) infection has better survival outcomes compared to non-HPV-related OPSCC, leading to efforts to de-escalate the intensity of treatment to reduce morbidity.
- Current de-escalation approaches in HPV-related OPSCC have focused on reducing or altering radiotherapy doses, systemic therapies, or incorporating neoadjuvant therapy.
- Transoral robotic surgery (TORS) is a minimally invasive surgical technique that has emerged as an additional treatment modality and potential component of treatment de-escalation regimens.
- Many recent and current clinical trials are exploring the role of TORS in de-escalation regimens, though none to date have demonstrated a consistent clinical benefit with respect to the current standard of care.

INTRODUCTION

Oropharyngeal squamous cell carcinoma (OPSCC) is the most common head and neck cancer in the United States. While it is historically associated with alcohol and tobacco use, there has been a recent increase in incidence due to its association with human papillomavirus (HPV) infection. It is estimated that over 30,000 cases of OPSCC will be diagnosed annually by 2030, the majority of which will be related to HPV.[1] Patients with HPV-related OPSCC are generally younger and healthier and do not have the same lifestyle risk factors.[2] Given this difference in presentation, optimizing treatment of this patient population has become an area of considerable research.

Department of Otolaryngology – Head and Neck Surgery, Vanderbilt University Medical Center, 1215 Medical Center Drive, Nashville, TN 27232, USA
* Corresponding author.
E-mail address: john.ceremsak@vumc.org

Surg Oncol Clin N Am 33 (2024) 697–709
https://doi.org/10.1016/j.soc.2024.07.001
1055-3207/24/© 2024 Elsevier Inc. All rights reserved, including those for text and data mining, AI training, and similar technologies.

The current treatment paradigm for HPV-related OPSCC was developed in an era in which the majority of OPSCC was related to alcohol and tobacco use. These non-HPV-related cases are associated with high rates of locoregional recurrence. Traditional treatment involves intense multimodal regimens consisting of surgery, radiation, and chemotherapy, often resulting in significant morbidity.[3] By contrast, HPV-related OPSCC exhibits improved sensitivity to radiation and chemotherapy and has much higher rates of locoregional control (LRC) and overall survival (OS).[4] Because of these excellent outcomes, attention has shifted toward focusing on reducing the morbidity of treatment. De-escalation, rather than intensification, has become the common theme of many clinical trials over the last decade.

Over this same period, minimally invasive surgical approaches such as transoral robotic surgery (TORS) and transoral laser microsurgery (TLM) have emerged as effective treatment modalities for oropharyngeal cancer. These technologies have become incorporated in the broader effort to de-escalate treatment intensity in HPV-related OPSCC. While surgery is not without its own risks, side effects, and toxicities, it does offer distinct advantages over primary chemoradiation. These include the ability to reduce gross tumor burden rapidly and provide more accurate staging and pathologic assessment.

The parallel push toward treatment de-escalation in HPV-related OPSCC and the emergence of TORS have resulted in a considerable opportunity to advance the treatment of this increasingly prevalent disease. This article reviews the clinical efforts made to de-escalate primary radiation therapy (RT) and chemoradiation therapy (CRT) in the treatment of HPV-related OPSCC and evaluate the role of TORS in achieving this aim.

PRIMARY CHEMORADIATION DE-ESCALATION STRATEGIES
Radiotherapy Dose Reduction

The most straightforward approach for treatment de-escalation in HPV-related OPSCC is to alter the dose and/or delivery of radiation to the primary tumor site with the objective of reducing side effects including xerostomia, dysphagia, and neck fibrosis. While standard doses used to treat OPSCC are roughly 70 Gy, doses below 60 Gy have been shown to be associated with improved swallowing function.[5] Several clinical trials have attempted to achieve this degree of reduction while maintaining acceptable oncologic outcomes. In 2015 and 2019, Chera and colleagues[6,7] reported single-institution results from phase II trials enrolling patients with both early and advanced (T0-T3, N0-N2) disease and found that a reduced dose of 60 Gy over 6 weeks when given with concurrent cisplatin resulted in 2 year LRC and OS rates of 86% and 95%, respectively. The studies reported favorable quality-of-life outcomes including swallowing function and xerostomia 1 year after treatment. Overall, the authors argued in favor of further exploring the role of reduced-dose RT, particularly in those with more favorable-risk diseases.

Other trials have investigated the efficacy of delivering a reduced dose of RT over an accelerated course while also omitting concurrent chemotherapy entirely. NRG HN002 enrolled patients with early and advanced (T1-T2 N1-N2b or T3 N0-N2) disease and randomized participants to receive either 60 Gy delivered over 6 weeks with concurrent cisplatin or 60 Gy delivered over 5 weeks without any concurrent chemotherapy.[8] Two year progression-free survival (PFS) rates were 91% in the CRT arm and 88% in the accelerated RT arm. Both arms had comparable OS above 95%. With respect to toxicity, the study identified more acute adverse events in the CRT arm but no difference in late adverse events or swallowing outcomes at 1 year.

Further modifications to both RT dose and systemic therapy are currently being explored in NRG HN005, a phase II/III study comparing disease control rates using reduced-dose RT (60 Gy) with cisplatin or the anti-programmed cell death 1 (PD-1) monoclonal antibody nivolumab against the standard of care (70 Gy with cisplatin). Of note, this study is currently closed to accrual as interim analysis demonstrated that the 60 Gy with cisplatin arm did not meet predesignated non-inferiority criteria compared to the standard-of-care arm.

As patients with HPV-related OPSCC are generally younger and healthier at diagnosis, the push to avoid long-term and late side effects by reducing RT doses to 60 Gy is an important component of the evolving treatment paradigm for HPV-related OPSCC. The question of whether these lower doses result in durable oncologic outcomes remains the subject of debate.

Replacement of Platinum-based Chemotherapy with Cetuximab

Traditional platinum-based chemotherapy can have significant side effects, particularly when used concurrently with radiotherapy. Over the last decade, efforts have been made to explore the replacement of cisplatin with the monoclonal anti-epidermal growth factor receptor (EGFR) antibody cetuximab. Cetuximab first emerged as a potential therapy in 2006 when Bonner and colleagues reported improved survival in patients with upper airway squamous cell carcinoma who underwent a cetuximab-based CRT regimen compared to those who underwent RT monotherapy.[9] Subsequent subgroup analysis showed this survival benefit was more pronounced in OPSCC as well as younger patients with better performance status, suggesting the therapy may be effective in HPV-related OPSCC.[10]

However, further clinical investigation has raised concerns about the effectiveness of cetuximab in CRT regimens. The RTOG 1016, De-ESCALaTE, ARTSCAN III, and TROG 12.01 trials all randomized patients with stage III or IV disease to receive either cetuximab or cisplatin in combination with standard RT and noted inferior LRC and decreased OS.[11–14] These studies suggested that either cisplatin is an important radiation sensitizer or that cetuximab is an inferior treatment. To date, preclinical data have not shown a radiosensitizing effect of cetuximab; by contrast, it has been shown that HPV-related OPSCC harbors fewer driver mutations and molecular alterations such as EGFR overexpression.[15] Perhaps most notably, these studies did not find a significant reduction in the incidence of moderate or severe adverse events in those receiving cetuximab. For these reasons, cisplatin has remained the standard-of-care systemic therapy used in CRT protocols, although further investigation in patients who are unable to tolerate cisplatin may be warranted.

Induction Chemotherapy or Immunotherapy Followed by Reduced Chemoradiation

The role of induction or neoadjuvant therapy has been explored in several clinical studies under the premise that a positive response to induction therapy can stratify patients by their likelihood to respond to reduced-intensity definitive therapy. In 2017, Chen and colleagues[16] reported the results of a single-arm phase II trial in which 44 patients with stage III and IV disease were given 2 cycles of an induction regimen consisting of paclitaxel and carboplatin and were subsequently assigned to either 54 or 60 Gy CRT depending on their initial response. Overall, 54% of enrolled patients achieved a partial or complete response and were assigned to the reduced-dose CRT arm; 2 year PFS in this group was 92%.

Marur and colleagues[17] subsequently reported the results of E1308, a similar phase II trial in which 80 patients with stage III and IV disease were given an induction regimen of cisplatin, paclitaxel, and cetuximab and then assigned to either 54 or 70 Gy, each with cetuximab, depending on their response. Overall, 70% of patients achieved a complete response and were treated with reduced dose RT and cetuximab. Two year PFS and OS in the reduced-dose arm were 80% and 94%, respectively; however, the authors noted that PFS and OS improved to 96% and 96%, respectively, when patients with T4 and N2c disease and greater than 10 pack-year smoking history were excluded. The study noted significantly less dysphagia and improved nutritional status at 1 year.

The OPTIMA trial sought to further reduce RT doses based on response to induction therapy. Patients were given an induction regimen of carboplatin and paclitaxel and responses were graded by Response Evaluation Criteria in Solid Tumors (RECIST) scores. Those with low-risk ($\leq$T3, $\leq$N2b, and $\leq$10 pack-year smoking history) disease with 50% or more response were assigned to 50 Gy RT monotherapy, while low-risk partial responders (<50% by RECIST) and high-risk patients with 50% or more response were assigned to 45 Gy CRT. Of the 61 patients who completed induction therapy, 20 received 50 Gy RT and 30 received 45 Gy CRT. Two year PFS for low-risk and high-risk patients was 95% and 94%, respectively. Severe mucositis occurred in 30% and 63% of the RT-only and CRT arms, respectively, compared to 91% in those assigned to the standard-of-care regimen of 75 Gy CRT. Percutaneous gastrostomy (PEG) tube use was 0% and 31% in the RT-only and CRT arms, respectively, compared to 82% in the standard-of-care arm.

More recently, the use of neoadjuvant immunotherapy has become the subject of clinical investigation. OPTIMA II, published in 2024, investigated the use of neoadjuvant regimen consisting of nivolumab and chemotherapy in patients with stage III or IV disease.[18] As in OPTIMA, patients were subsequently assigned to treatment arms based on response and risk status. Of the 73 patients who completed induction, 51 (71%) experienced 50% or more response by RECIST. Sixty-two patients (86%) ultimately received reduced-intensity therapy with 50 Gy RT monotherapy, surgery, or a reduced 45 to 50 Gy CRT regimen. Those who received RT monotherapy or underwent surgery had 2 year PFS and OS of 96% and 96%, respectively. Those who underwent reduced-dose CRT had 2 year PFS and OS of 88% and 91%, respectively. Both groups were noted to have better functional outcomes including improved swallowing and a lower rate of enteral feeding. Notably, the improvement in PFS was more pronounced in those with programmed death-ligand 1 expression, suggesting it may serve as a useful biomarker in future studies investigating the use of immunotherapy.

SURGICAL DE-ESCALATION STRATEGIES: TRANSORAL ROBOTIC SURGERY
Patient Selection, Technique, and Surgical Morbidity

Historically, surgical approaches for the treatment of OPSCC were highly invasive, often requiring lip-split mandibulotomy for adequate exposure and complex reconstruction. These procedures were associated with frequent perioperative complications and long-term morbidities.[19] For this reason, the treatment paradigm for OPSCC gradually shifted to one favoring primary chemoradiation.[20] Over the past 15 years, however, the emergence of minimally invasive techniques such as TORS and TLM has reintroduced surgery as a treatment modality that can help achieve comparable oncologic outcomes while preserving key physiologic functions such as swallowing.[21,22,23]

The principles of all minimally invasive surgical approaches, including TORS, involve maximizing exposure while minimizing morbidity to achieve a complete oncologic resection with the smallest safe negative margin possible. Central to this aim is appropriate patient selection. Patients with advanced or endophytic oropharyngeal disease with involvement of critical soft tissue or vascular structures are less amenable to a TORS approach.[24] Moreover, TORS carries additional short-term risks of bleeding, airway compromise, and dehydration. Patients must be appropriately counseled and be of a certain functional status to withstand these potential issues in the immediate postoperative period.

Morbidity associated with TORS for OPSCC can broadly be categorized into short-term and long-term effects. Weinstein and colleagues[25] performed a multicenter retrospective review of 177 patients who previously underwent TORS and found that the most common adverse events were acute dysphagia (9%) and oral bleeding requiring operative control (3%). Elective tracheostomy was performed in 22 patients (12%) but all but 4 were decannulated by 1 year after surgery. The rate of PEG tube use in those who had not received any prior RT was 5%. More recent single-institution data from Van Abel and colleagues found lower rates of both tracheostomy (6%) and PEG tube use (3%), suggesting that surgeons may have been initially overly aggressive in pursuing these interventions when TORS was first introduced.[26]

Once patients transition from the immediate postoperative period, longer term morbidity associated with TORS reflects the surgical alteration of the anatomy of the upper airway resulting in swallowing, speech, and respiratory issues. If surgery is to be considered a viable treatment modality in HPV-related OPSCC, this long-term morbidity must not simply replace the improvements realized by de-escalation of RT and CRT, a concept referred to as toxicity equipoise.[27] This concept was first investigated in the ORATOR study, which randomized patients with low-to-intermediate risk (T1–T2, N0–2) disease to 70 Gy RT or TORS with neck dissection (ND) and adjuvant therapy as indicated. The primary outcome was dysphagia as reported by medical doctor (MD) Anderson Dysphagia Inventory scores.[28] The study reported that superior swallowing outcomes were associated with primary RT, though the difference did not reflect a clinically significant change. A prospective longitudinal study performed at MD Anderson investigated swallowing outcomes in those with low-to-intermediate risk (T1–T3, N0–2b) disease treated either with upfront TORS or intensity-modulated proton therapy and found that dysphagia as graded by Dynamic Imaging Grade for Swallowing Toxicty scores favored upfront TORS at 3 to 6 months postoperatively.[29] Taken together, these data support that dysphagia following TORS is at least comparable to that seen after primary RT or CRT. While the length of follow-up is limited in both studies, these results may favor the superiority of surgical intervention as RT-associated dysphagia has been shown to progress with time.[30]

Randomized Trials Comparing Primary RT or CRT with Transoral Robotic Surgery

To date, it remains unclear whether a primary surgical or RT-based approach is superior for the treatment of HPV-related OPSCC. The ORATOR study, described earlier, was the first study to directly compare these approaches; however, the primary endpoint was swallowing outcomes rather than progression or survival as the study included non-HPV-related OPSCC and was not designed to compare any de-escalation treatment regimens. ORATOR2, a follow-up study to ORATOR, was designed to address these questions of de-escalation and survival. In a multicenter phase II randomized trial, the study enrolled patients with HPV-related OPSCC (T1-2, N0-2) to arms consisting of primary 60 Gy CRT or primary TORS and ND with adjuvant therapy based on pathologic findings.[31] Patients who underwent TORS and were found to have extranodal extension (ENE) or positive margins received 60 Gy adjuvant RT, while those with close margins (<3 mm), multiple nodes, large nodes (>3 cm), lymphovascular invasion (LVI), perineural invasion (PNI), or advanced disease (pT3–4) received 50 Gy adjuvant RT. Of 31 patients assigned to TORS and ND, 21 (78%) received adjuvant therapy with a median dose of 52 Gy. The study was halted due to adverse events in the surgical arm, including 2 treatment-related deaths. The authors concluded that surgery should be recommended with caution; however, survival data have yet to be reported.

Additional trials are actively investigating direct comparisons of primary RT versus surgery. The "best of" trial (NCT02984410) and (Quality of Life After Primary TORS vs IMRT for Patients With Early-stage Oropharyngeal Squamous Cell Carcinoma [QoLATI]) trial (NCT04124198) are both phase III studies registered in Europe which are enrolling patients with early-stage (T1-2, N0-1) disease with assignment to accelerated RT (66–70 Gy) or surgery with adjuvant therapy as indicated. Like (a Phase II Randomized Trial for Early-Stage Squamous Cell Carcinoma of the Oropharynx: Radiotherapy vs Transoral Robotic Surgery [ORATOR]), the primary endpoint for these studies is swallowing outcomes rather than survival. It should be noted the "best of" study includes additional anatomic subsites beyond the oropharynx and allows for multiple surgical approaches including TLM or conventional transoral surgery. Each study should help further elucidate the safety and important quality-of-life metrics associated with primary surgery.

Radiotherapy Dose Reduction after Transoral Robotic Surgery

As clinical studies continue to investigate the safety and morbidity associated with TORS, parallel studies are exploring the use of reduced adjuvant therapy in postoperative patients (**Table 1**).[32] Among the first to report on this de-escalation strategy was the single-arm phase II A Phase 2 Trial of Alternative Volumes of Oropharyngeal Irradiation for De-intensificationSIRS: Sinai Robotic Surgery (AVOID) trial in which patients who previously underwent TORS and were found to have favorable-risk pathology (negative margins, no LVI or PNI) were not given adjuvant RT to the primary site.[33] Sixty patients were enrolled with 2 year PFS and OS of 92.1% and 100%, respectively, suggesting more limited adjuvant radiation may be feasible in selected patients.

The phase II sinai robotic surgery (SIRS) trial evaluated RT de-intensification after TORS resection with stratification based on pathologic risk factors.[34] Those with intermediate-risk (LVI, PNI, or ≤ 1 mm ENE) or high-risk (ENE, positive margins, >3 positive lymph nodes) features were assigned to adjuvant regimens of 50 Gy RT and 56 Gy CRT, respectively. Fifty-four patients were enrolled; 2 year PFS rates in the intermediate-risk and high-risk arms were 87% and 93%, respectively.

Eastern cooperative oncology group (ECOG) 3311 was a phase II study, similar to SIRS, which evaluated adjuvant therapy based on pathologic findings.[35] In contrast to SIRS, the intermediate-risk arm was expanded to include those with close margins (≤ 3 mm) and large (>3 cm) positive lymph nodes and those randomized patients with intermediate-risk features to either 50 or 60 Gy adjuvant RT. The study reported 2 year PFS of 95% and 96% in these 2 arms, respectively, but noted an improved side effect profile in the 50 Gy cohort. Because of these promising findings, ECOG is planning a phase III study to compare their 50 Gy RT approach with the current standard of care.

The (a phase II/III trial of risk-stratified, reduced intensity adjuvant treatment in patients undergoing transoral surgery for human papillomavirus [HPV]-positive oropharyngeal cancer [PATHOS]) trial is an ongoing phase II/III randomized controlled trial registered in the United Kingdom that aims to study adjuvant treatment de-intensification with primary outcome measures of long-term swallowing function and OS.[36] Treatment arms are stratified by pathologic assessment into intermediate-risk (60 Gy vs 50 Gy) and high-risk (60 Gy with cisplatin vs 60 Gy RT monotherapy) groups. Results of this trial have not yet been published.

Table 1
Clinical trials investigating survival with de-escalated adjuvant therapy following upfront TORS in HPV-related OPSCC

Year	Trial	Key Inclusion Criteria[a]	Experimental Treatment Arm(s)	Outcomes
2019	AVOID (NCT02159703)	pT1-2 >2 mm margins No PNI or LVI	Single arm: No adjuvant RT to primary site	• 2 y LRC 97.9%, OS 100%
2019	MC1273 (NCT01932697)	Stage III-IV ≤10 pack-year smoking ≥1 of: pT3, LN >3 cm, 2+ LN, PNI/LVI, ENE	A: ≥T4, ≥N2, LVI or PNI: 30 Gy CRT B: Any ENE: 36 Gy CRT	• A&B 2 y LRC 96.2%, PFS 91.1%, OS 98.7%
2021	MC1675 (DART-HPV) (NCT02908477)	Stage III-IV ≤10 pack-year smoking ≥1 of: pT3, LN >3 cm, 2+ LN, PNI/LVI, ENE	A: ≥T4, ≥N2, LVI or PNI: 30 Gy CRT B: Any ENE: 36 Gy CRT	• A&B 2 y LRC 95.5%, PFS 86.5%, OS 96.1% • A&B less toxic, improved QoL compared to standard of care
2022	SIRS (NCT02072148)	T1-2, N0-2b <20 pack-year smoking	A: T1-2, N1-2b, no ENE, LVI or PNI: Observe B: ≤1 mm ENE, LVI or PNI: 50 Gy RT C: Positive margins, ENE, 3+ nodes: 56 Gy CRT	• A 2 y PFS 91.3% • B 2 y PFS 86.7% • C 2 y PFS 93.3%
2022	E3311 (NCT01898494)	Stage III, IVa, IVb No radiographic ENE or matted nodes	A: T1-2, N0-1, no ENE: Observe B: T1-2 close margin, N1-2, ≤1 mm ENE: 50 Gy C: T1-2 close margin, N1-2, ≤1 mm ENE: 60 Gy D: Positive margins, >1 mm ENE: 66 Gy CRT	• A 2 y PFS 96.9% • B 2 y PFS 94.9% • C 2 y PFS 96.0% • D 2 y PFS 90.7%
2024	30 ROC - Phase II (NCT03323463)	T0-2, N1-2c Negative or microscopic positive margins	A: FMISO PET Non-hypoxic: 30 Gy CRT B: FMISO PET Hypoxic: 70 Gy CRT	• A 2 y PFS 94%, OS 100% • B 2 y PFS 96%, OS 96%

(continued on next page)

Table 1
(continued)

Year	Trial	Key Inclusion Criteria[a]	Experimental Treatment Arm(s)	Outcomes
-	PATHOS (NCT02215265)	T1-3, N0-2b ≤10 pack-year smoking	A: T1-2, N0-1: Observe B1: T3, N2, close margin, LVI or PNI: 50 Gy B2: T3, N2, close margin, LVI or PNI: ˆ0 Gy C1: Positive margins, ENE: 60 Gy RT C2: Positive margins, ENE: 60 Gy CRT	N/A

[a] AJCC 7th ed. criteria.

In addition to radiation de-intensification alone, combination therapy with the addition of systemic agents may allow for greater decreases in RT dose while preserving outcomes. Ma and colleagues[37] investigated aggressive RT de-escalation in combination with docetaxel after surgical resection in a single arm phase II trial (MC1273). Patients with intermediate-risk features were assigned to 30 Gy CRT with docetaxel, while those with high-risk features (positive ENE) were assigned to 36 Gy CRT with docetaxel. In the aggregate 80 patient cohort, survival outcomes that were comparable to other studies with a 2 year PFS were 91% and OS of 99%. With respect to toxicities, there study noted significant improvements in each arm compared to the standard of care, suggesting that even triple-modality therapy, when reduced appropriately, can achieve good outcomes with reduced morbidity. Given these promising results, a follow-up phase III trial is currently underway (DART-HPV, NCT02908477) that plans to randomize patients to compare this regimen with the standard-of-care.

Additional studies are investigating the use of immunotherapy in lieu of adjuvant systemic therapy. Skinner and colleagues[38] reported the results of a phase II trial that sought to de-escalate RT dose with the addition of nivolumab. Patients with pathologic stage III or IVa HPV-associated OPSCC with high-risk features (ENE, ≥ 5 positive lymph nodes) were treated with 50 Gy with concurrent nivolumab. Three year PFS and OS in this cohort were 86% and 97%, respectively, suggesting that RT de-escalation in conjunction with immunotherapy may be a viable de-escalation approach in patients who previously underwent TORS.

Most recently, studies have begun to utilize novel approaches for postoperative risk stratification. In 2024, Lee and colleagues reported a single-institution phase II trial (which followed the pilot 30 ROC trial) that investigated aggressive de-escalation of RT doses to 30 Gy in patients who were found to have non-hypoxic tumors on postoperative ^{18}F-fluoromisonidazole PET imaging.[39,40] Of 152 enrolled patients, 128 (84%) ultimately received the reduced dose of 30 Gy and were found to have 2 year LRS and PFS rates of 94.7% and 94%, respectively.

De-escalation Informed by Surgical Pathology

The current diagnostic approach for HPV-related OPSCC relies on clinical examination, radiographic evaluation, and tissue biopsy often via fine-needle aspiration of a cervical lymph node. Certain disease factors, including tumor invasiveness, margin status, number of involved lymph nodes, and ENE, have all been shown as predictors of improved response to a de-escalated treatment plan. For example, traditional imaging has been shown to inconsistently detect the presence of ENE, with sensitivity and specificity near 60% and 75%, respectively.[41] As new studies continue to identify biomarkers and genetic alterations that may serve provide additional prognostic information, there has emerged a need to obtain adequate tissue sampling early in the treatment course. While this remains a rapidly evolving area of research, there is reason to believe that upfront surgical intervention and its ability to provide more comprehensive pathologic data represent an advantage beyond simply reducing disease burden in anticipation of adjuvant therapy.

FUTURE DIRECTIONS

The evolution of the treatment paradigm for HPV-related OPSCC reflects a fortunate reality that patients are more likely to experience long-term survival, thus shifting the focus from improving mortality to reducing the morbidity associated with treatment. A variety of frameworks for de-escalation of the current standard for CRT have been proposed and TORS has emerged as a valuable third treatment modality, widening the scope of potential regimens that could ultimately be used to preserve survival while reducing treatment morbidity. However, these de-escalation strategies remain largely dependent on clinical staging, smoking status, response to systemic therapy, or, in the case of surgical cases, pathologic features. The development of novel imaging protocols and molecular tests will help to more appropriately risk-stratify patients, particularly those undergoing upfront surgical intervention, to personalize adjuvant therapy. Perhaps most promising among these is the development of assays to detect circulating tumor DNA that has been shown to complement imaging in the detection of residual disease and postoperatively is associated with the progression of disease and worse OS.[42,43]

SUMMARY

Given the excellent survival outcomes of patients with HPV-related OPSCC treated with standard-of-care regimens, surgery alone is unlikely to replace definitive CRT as a primary treatment modality. As further efforts are made to identify patient-specific factors that predict a favorable disease profile, however, TORS is poised to play a central role in permitting significant de-escalation of adjuvant therapy and improving quality of life without compromising disease progression or survival. Efforts to de-escalate radiation and chemotherapy regimens have been consistently successful in studies employing upfront surgery but less so in those without surgical therapy. This produces a dilemma, as the long-term morbidity of surgery with reduced adjuvant therapy versus nonsurgical therapy alone is not yet defined.

CLINICS CARE POINTS

- Patients with OPSCC related to HPV infection likely benefit from decreased treatment intensity as it has been should to reduce treatment-related morbidity while maintaining excellent oncologic outcomes.
- TORS is a potentially useful treatment modality in select patients with OPSCC.
- Currently, there is no definitive evidence that de-escalation therapy involving TORS provides an advantage over de-escalation regimens involving traditional chemoradiation.

DISCLOSURE

The authors have nothing to disclose.

REFERENCES

1. Tota JE, Best AF, Zumsteg ZS, et al. Evolution of the oropharynx cancer epidemic in the United States: moderation of increasing incidence in younger individuals and shift in the burden to older individuals. J Clin Oncol 2019;37(18). JCO.1 9.00370.
2. Pytynia KB, Dahlstrom KR, Sturgis EM. Epidemiology of HPV-associated oropharyngeal cancer. Oral Oncol 2014;50(5):380–6.
3. Machtay M, Moughan J, Trotti A, et al. Factors associated with severe late toxicity after concurrent chemoradiation for locally advanced head and neck cancer: an RTOG analysis. J Clin Oncol 2008;26(21):3582–9.
4. Ang KK, Jonathan H, Richard W, et al. Human Papillomavirus And Survival Of Patients With Oropharyngeal Cancer. N Engl J Med 2010;363(1):24–35.

5. Mortensen HR, Jensen K, Aksglæde K, et al. Late dysphagia after IMRT for head and neck cancer and correlation with dose-volume parameters. Radiother Oncol J Eur Soc Ther Radiol Oncol 2013;107(3):288–94.

6. Chera BS, Amdur RJ, Tepper J, et al. Phase 2 trial of de-intensified chemoradiation therapy for favorable-risk human papillomavirus–associated oropharyngeal squamous cell carcinoma. Int J Radiat Oncol 2015;93(5):976–85.

7. Chera BS, Amdur RJ, Green R, et al. Phase II trial of de-intensified chemoradiotherapy for human papillomavirus–associated oropharyngeal squamous cell carcinoma. J Clin Oncol 2019;37(29):2661–9.

8. Yom SS, Torres-Saavedra P, Caudell JJ, et al. Reduced-dose radiation therapy for hpv-associated oropharyngeal carcinoma (NRG Oncology HN002). J Clin Oncol 2021;39(9):956–65.

9. Bonner JA, Harari PM, Giralt J, et al. Radiotherapy plus cetuximab for squamous-cell carcinoma of the head and neck. N Engl J Med 2006;354(6):567–78.

10. Bonner JA, Harari PM, Giralt J, et al. Radiotherapy plus cetuximab for locoregionally advanced head and neck cancer: 5-year survival data from a phase 3 randomised trial, and relation between cetuximab-induced rash and survival. Lancet Oncol 2010;11(1):21–8.

11. Gillison ML, Trotti AM, Harris J, et al. Radiotherapy plus cetuximab or cisplatin in human papillomavirus-positive oropharyngeal cancer (NRG Oncology RTOG 1016): a randomised, multicentre, non-inferiority trial. Lancet 2019;393(10166): 40–50.

12. Mehanna H, Robinson M, Hartley A, et al. Radiotherapy plus cisplatin or cetuximab in low-risk human papillomavirus-positive oropharyngeal cancer (De-ESCA-LaTE HPV): an open-label randomised controlled phase 3 trial. Lancet 2019; 393(10166):51–60.

13. Rischin D, King M, Kenny L, et al. Randomized trial of radiation therapy with weekly cisplatin or cetuximab in low-risk HPV-associated oropharyngeal cancer (TROG 12.01) – a trans-tasman radiation oncology group study. Int J Radiat Oncol 2021;111(4):876–86.

14. Gebre-Medhin M, Brun E, Engström P, et al. ARTSCAN III: a randomized phase iii study comparing chemoradiotherapy with cisplatin versus cetuximab in patients with locoregionally advanced head and neck squamous cell cancer. J Clin Oncol 2021;39(1):38–47.

15. Mirghani H, Amen F, Moreau F, et al. Oropharyngeal cancers: Relationship between epidermal growth factor receptor alterations and human papillomavirus status. Eur J Cancer 2014;50(6):1100–11.

16. Chen AM, Felix C, Wang PC, et al. Reduced-dose radiotherapy for human papillomavirus-associated squamous-cell carcinoma of the oropharynx: a single-arm, phase 2 study. Lancet Oncol 2017;18(6):803–11.

17. Marur S, Li S, Cmelak AJ, et al. E1308: Phase II trial of induction chemotherapy followed by reduced-dose radiation and weekly cetuximab in patients with HPV-associated resectable squamous cell carcinoma of the oropharynx— ECOG-ACRIN cancer research group. J Clin Oncol 2016;35(5):490–7.

18. Rosenberg AJ, Agrawal N, Juloori A, et al. Neoadjuvant nivolumab plus chemotherapy followed by response-adaptive therapy for HPV+ oropharyngeal cancer: OPTIMA II phase 2 open-label nonrandomized controlled trial. JAMA Oncol 2024; 10(7):923–31.

19. Dziegielewski PT, Mlynarek AM, Dimitry J, et al. The mandibulotomy: Friend or foe? Safety outcomes and literature review. Laryngoscope 2009;119(12): 2369–75.

20. Chen AY, Schrag N, Hao Y, et al. Changes in treatment of advanced oropharyngeal cancer, 1985–2001. Laryngoscope 2007;117(1):16–21.
21. Moore EJ, Abel KMV, Price DL, et al. Transoral robotic surgery for oropharyngeal carcinoma: Surgical margins and oncologic outcomes. Head Neck 2018;40(4): 747–55.
22. Moore EJ, Olsen SM, Laborde RR, et al. Long-term functional and oncologic results of transoral robotic surgery for oropharyngeal squamous cell carcinoma. Mayo Clin Proc 2012;87(3):219–25.
23. Rich JT, Milov S, Lewis JS, et al. Transoral laser microsurgery (TLM) ± adjuvant therapy for advanced stage oropharyngeal cancer. Laryngoscope 2009;119(9): 1709–19.
24. Baskin RM, Boyce BJ, Amdur R, et al. Transoral robotic surgery for oropharyngeal cancer: patient selection and special considerations. Cancer Manag Res 2018; 10:839–46.
25. Weinstein GS, O'Malley BW, Magnuson JS, et al. Transoral robotic surgery: a multicenter study to assess feasibility, safety, and surgical margins. Laryngoscope 2012;122(8):1701–7.
26. Abel KMV, Quick MH, Graner DE, et al. Outcomes following TORS for HPV-positive oropharyngeal carcinoma: PEGs, tracheostomies, and beyond. Am J Otolaryngol 2019;40(5):729–34.
27. Ma DJ, Abel KMV. Treatment De-intensification for HPV-associated Oropharyngeal Cancer: A Definitive Surgery Paradigm. Semin Radiat Oncol 2021;31(4): 332–8.
28. Nichols AC, Theurer J, Prisman E, et al. Radiotherapy versus transoral robotic surgery and neck dissection for oropharyngeal squamous cell carcinoma (ORATOR): an open-label, phase 2, randomised trial. Lancet Oncol 2019;20(10) :1349–59.
29. Barbon CE, Peterson CB, Dirba DD, et al. Comparison of prospective, longitudinal swallowing function after primary intensity-modulated proton therapy (IMPT) or transoral robotic surgery (TORS) for oropharyngeal squamous cell carcinoma. Int J Radiat Oncol 2020;108(3):S160.
30. Embring A, Onjukka E, Mercke C, et al. Dose escalation of oropharyngeal cancer: long-time follow-up and side effects. Cancers 2023;15(9):2580.
31. Palma DA, Prisman E, Berthelet E, et al. Assessment of toxic effects and survival in treatment deescalation with radiotherapy vs transoral surgery for HPV-associated oropharyngeal squamous cell carcinoma. JAMA Oncol 2022; 8(6):1–7.
32. Mirghani H, Blanchard P. Treatment de-escalation for HPV-driven oropharyngeal cancer: Where do we stand? Clin Transl Radiat Oncol 2018;8:4–11.
33. Swisher-McClure S, Lukens JN, Aggarwal C, et al. A phase 2 trial of alternative volumes of oropharyngeal irradiation for de-intensification (AVOID): omission of the resected primary tumor bed after transoral robotic surgery for human papilloma virus–related squamous cell carcinoma of the oropharynx. Int J Radiat Oncol 2020;106(4):725–32.
34. Miles BA, Posner MR, Gupta V, et al. De-escalated adjuvant therapy after transoral robotic surgery for human papillomavirus-related oropharyngeal carcinoma: the sinai robotic surgery (SIRS) Trial. Oncol 2021;26(6):504–13.
35. Ferris RL, Flamand Y, Weinstein GS, et al. Phase II randomized trial of transoral surgery and low-dose intensity modulated radiation therapy in resectable p16+ locally advanced oropharynx cancer: an ECOG-ACRIN cancer research group trial (E3311). J Clin Oncol 2022;40(2):138–49.

36. Hargreaves S, Beasley M, Hurt C, et al. Deintensification of adjuvant treatment after transoral surgery in patients with human papillomavirus-positive oropharyngeal cancer: the conception of the PATHOS study and its development. Front Oncol 2019;9:936.
37. Ma DJ, Price KA, Moore EJ, et al. Phase II evaluation of aggressive dose de-escalation for adjuvant chemoradiotherapy in human papillomavirus–associated oropharynx squamous cell carcinoma. J Clin Oncol 2019;37(22):1909–18.
38. Skinner HD, Zandberg DP, Raben A, et al. Phase II trial of adjuvant de-escalated radiation + adjuvant nivolumab for intermediate-high risk P16+ oropharynx cancer. J Clin Oncol 2023;41(16_suppl):6014.
39. Riaz N, Sherman E, Pei X, et al. Precision radiotherapy: reduction in radiation for oropharyngeal cancer in the 30 ROC trial. JNCI J Natl Cancer Inst 2021;113(6):742–51.
40. Lee NY, Sherman EJ, Schöder H, et al. Hypoxia-directed treatment of human papillomavirus–related oropharyngeal carcinoma. J Clin Oncol 2024;42(8):940–50.
41. Carlton JA, Maxwell AW, Bauer LB, et al. Computed tomography detection of extracapsular spread of squamous cell carcinoma of the head and neck in metastatic cervical lymph nodes. NeuroRadiol J 2017;30(3):222–9.
42. Rutkowski TW, Mazurek AM, Śnietura M, et al. Circulating HPV16 DNA may complement imaging assessment of early treatment efficacy in patients with HPV-positive oropharyngeal cancer. J Transl Med 2020;18(1):167.
43. Routman DM, Chera BS, Jethwa KR, et al. Detectable HPV ctDNA in post-operative oropharyngeal squamous cell carcinoma patients is associated with progression. Int J Radiat Oncol 2019;105(3):682–3.

State of Head and Neck Microvascular Reconstruction
Current and Future Directions

Michael M. Li, MD, Lauren E. Miller, MD, MBA, Matthew Old, MD*

KEYWORDS

- Head and neck • Microvascular reconstruction • Free flap • Advances

KEY POINTS

- Microvascular free tissue transfer (MFTT) has become more prevalent and complex, without compromise in flap or patient survival.
- Patient and flap selection for MFTT is guided in large part by the need to reconstruct a defect following an oncologically sound ablation.
- Technological advances including medical modeling, 3-D printing, and advanced imaging will continue to improve oncologic and reconstructive outcomes.

BACKGROUND

Over the past decades, head and neck microvascular reconstruction has undergone major advances. Accordingly, microvascular free tissue transfer (MFTT) has become more prevalent and complex, without compromise in flap or patient survival. Contemporary free tissue transfer success rates often exceed 95%.[1–3] With high success rates and improving head and neck cancer survival, new challenges in microvascular reconstruction have arisen, demanding a focus on novel techniques, improved functional outcomes, and the application of developing technologies.[4] In this review, the authors address the current state of microvascular reconstruction with a focus on advancements across the perioperative course. The authors additionally discuss future directions in free flap reconstruction and techniques.

PREOPERATIVE
Patient Selection

Patient and flap selection for MFTT is guided in large part by the need to reconstruct a defect following an oncologically sound ablation. In recent years, factors such as

Department of Otolaryngology Head and Neck Surgery, Ohio State University James Cancer Center, 460 West 10th Avenue, Columbus, OH 43210, USA
* Corresponding author.
E-mail address: matthew.old@osumc.edu

Surg Oncol Clin N Am 33 (2024) 711–721
https://doi.org/10.1016/j.soc.2024.04.004
1055-3207/24/© 2024 Elsevier Inc. All rights reserved.

surgonc.theclinics.com

expanding donor site options, improved surgical outcomes, decreased operative times, and an increasing need to address survivorship-related concerns have expanded the patient population for MFTT. Further expanding the MFTT population is the fact that success rates have remained high despite significant comorbidities in the head and neck patient population such as active smoking, cardiovascular disease, and uncontrolled diabetes. Additionally, while elderly age (defined variably as >65, 75, or 80 years old) at the time of surgery is associated with increased rates of perioperative medical complications, several studies have demonstrated no difference in flap survival rates in elderly patients as compared to younger patients.[5–7] As the overall population has aged, head and neck surgeons will be required to manage and operate on an increasingly sicker populace. Additionally, as the overall patient population ages and survival improves, surgery may increasingly become necessary to address survivorship and functional-related concerns such as osteoradionecrosis, dysphagia, chronic fistula, and cosmetic concerns. Balancing a given patient's risk of anesthesia and associated comorbidities with the benefit of undergoing MFTT with increasing survivorship is an increasingly important component of the head and neck cancer surgeon preoperative workup.

Incorporating Enhanced Recovery After Surgery into Preoperative Patient Care

The Enhanced Recovery After Surgery (ERAS) Society has published guidelines on optimal care of head and neck cancer patients undergoing surgery. In 2016, consensus guidelines for patients undergoing major head and neck surgery and free flap reconstruction were released.[8] Drawing upon systematic reviews and findings primarily from studies of thoracic and abdominal surgeries, the guidelines provided recommendations for the use of preoperative carbohydrate nutrition, pharmacologic thromboprophylaxis, intraoperative antibiotic use, goal-directed fluid management, opioid-sparing analgesia, early postoperative mobilization, and the avoidance of perioperative fasting.

While many academic institutions currently incorporate components of ERAS, future steps in enhancing recovery may include preoperative rehabilitation (pre-habilitation). In one study of patients undergoing major abdominal or head and neck surgery, a 7-day pre-habilitation regimen consisting of increased physical activity, a carbohydrate drink, incentive spirometry, and chlorhexidine gluconate bath resulted in improved postoperative mobilization and decreased rates of pulmonary complications.[9] Studies of patients undergoing care for prostate, breast, and lung cancer have also shown directed pre-habilitation exercises decrease postoperative length of stay and rate of perioperative complications.[10] Further, psychologic-focused pre-habilitation in breast and prostate cancer patients demonstrated improved mood, physical well-being, immune function, and sense of optimism.[10] Particularly relevant to head and neck cancer patients, dysphagia-targeted pre-habilitation, consisting of exercises overseen by a speech and language pathologist, has been shown to improve functional postoperative swallowing outcomes including improved taste, smell, mouth opening, salivary function, and maintenance of diet.[11] Dysphagia targeted pre-habilitation also has the potential to enhance outcomes for patients undergoing primary chemoradiation treatment. As high postoperative rehabilitation needs and depression in head and neck cancer patients have been identified as significant causes of mortality, psychological and physical pre-habilitation warrants further investigation.[12] By nature, all pre-habilitation regimens can be time and resource intensive and rely on patient compliance, potentially limiting their efficacy. Larger scale studies with standardized protocols may provide further evidence and support for pre-habilitation in the head and neck cancer population.

Immunonutrition, or an immune-enhancing preoperative diet, is a component of ERAS care that may improve postoperative outcomes in head and neck cancer patients. The goal of immunonutrition is to focus on a diet that supplies macronutrients to meet demand and nutrients that minimize mediators of inflammation.[13] A prior study utilized a shake providing 17g of protein and enriched in omega-3 fatty acids, arginine, and RNA nucleotides, consumed three times daily for 5 days preoperatively. Patients in this cohort demonstrated fewer postoperative complications as well as shorter hospital stays.[14] Interventions such as this hold promise for feasibility and preoperative preparation for a patient population that, generally speaking, is malnourished, ultimately contributing to postoperative wound complications.

Surgery for Survivorship-Related Concerns

Among the most common survivorship-related concerns in the head and neck population is lymphedema. Lymphedema supermicrosurgery, in which a lymph vessel is anastomosed to a vein or lymph nodes are transplanted to the lymphedema bed, has been shown to improve quality of life for breast cancer patients.[15] Although data supporting lymphedema microsurgery in the head and neck cancer is limited, case reports and series have shown promising results.[16] Similarly, in cases where 1 or both internal jugular veins (IJV) have been sacrificed, reconstruction of the IJV via anastomosis of the superior IJV stump to a distal recipient vessel (eg,: external jugular vein) can provide similar relief of lymphedema symptoms.[17]

Osteoradionecrosis (ORN) of the jaw (ORNJ) affects up to 15% of patients who receive radiation as part of therapy for head and neck cancer. Traditionally, microvascular reconstruction for ORNJ has been fraught with increased rates of surgical complications. However, severe ORN that limits function necessitates MFTT. In this setting, long-term intravenous antibiotics, guided by cultures taken from the remaining healthy bone, may reduce postoperative complication rates.[18]

Surgical Planning: Vessel-Depleted Necks

Of course, a major survivorship concern lies in recurrence and the need for reoperation. In this setting, wherein patients have previously undergone multi-modality treatment, MFTT can be complicated by various factors including decreased availability of donor vessels. Approximately 7% of patients with head and neck cancer undergoing MFTT present with a vessel-depleted neck.[19] Preoperative investigation can be helpful in the form of computed tomography (CT) angiography of the neck to understand options, laterality of neck exploration, and the need for pedicle length. Prior literature has highlighted moderate concordance between CT angiography findings of vessels available and surgical findings when evaluating for neck vessels.[20]

Even if vessels are available, radiation changes or tumor recurrence may render them prohibitive for use. In these scenarios, the use of vessels from untreated areas may be optimal. The transverse cervical artery and vein are vessels easily accessible in the lower neck and frequently outside of the field of radiation or surgical resection. Similarly, the internal mammary vessels are anatomically consistent vascular options for vessel-depleted necks with reliable flow.[19,21] Other arterial options from the thoracoacromial system are also viable.[22,23]

Once vessels are found, sometimes pedicle length can be insufficient given the altered anatomy and vessel course. In this scenario, interposition vein grafts can be used. Prior literature evaluated 91 patients with either a saphenous, cephalic, external jugular, or facial vein graft used with an average vein graft harvest length of 18 cm and used for both arterial and venous anastomosis.[24] While flap survival in this cohort was 85%, the study population had high rates of prior treatment, necessitating the use of vein grafts and potentially contributing to flap failure. Other studies have suggested vein grafts have no bearing on overall flap success rates.[25] It is likely that, when performed with rigorous surgical technique, vein grafts themselves have no bearing on overall flap success rates. Rather, it is the fact that vein grafts are needed in complex revision reconstructions that leads to potentially higher flap complication rates.

Surgical Planning: Medical Modeling

Three-dimensional (3-D)medical modeling is an increasingly used reconstructive adjunct in maxillary and mandibular lesions that uses computed tomography (CT) scan to pre-plan resection and bony reconstruction. Often, this includes preoperatively creating pre-bent or custom-milled reconstruction plates that allow for near-perfect contouring to a patient's native skeleton. Medical modeling also allows for patient-specific cutting guides and templates to promote accurate osteotomies, additionally easing the preplanned reconstruction. This preoperative modeling simplifies intraoperative decision-making, reduces operative time, and is generally preferred in complex midface cases.[26–28] Medical modeling improves bone to bone contact, with minimal deviation between planned and actual reconstruction amongst a cohort of 26 cases.[26,29] In one study, virtual medical modeling for 9 maxillary defects with scapula composite reconstruction resulted in quicker return to oral diet, lower incidence of hardware exposure hardware, and lower risk of enophthalmos.[30]

While not routinely completed currently, medical modeling also has the potential to map vascular anatomy such as the flap pedicle and cutaneous perforators.[31] This use of medical modeling allows for more accurate surgical planning and can guide flap trimming or skin paddle division. Similarly, preoperative imaging of the thigh for anterolateral thigh flaps can map perforator anatomy and determine angiosomes, thereby guiding decision-making, reducing operative time, and influencing choice of leg for flap harvest.[32]

Beyond improved operative time, multidisciplinary teams can better surgically plan using preoperative medical modeling; for example, inclusion of a prosthodontist or oral surgeon at the time of the virtual planning facilitates preplanning the sites of osseointegration for dental implants in patients undergoing dental restoration.[28,33] Finally, 3-D printed models are helpful for trainee education, allowing for preoperative discussion of the defect and reconstruction plan in a visual, interactive manner[29] (**Fig. 1**).

INTRAOPERATIVE

In the following section, the authors review and assess currently used medications, surgical techniques, and technologies with an eye toward the future.

Intraoperative Medications

Aside from the near consensus use of aspirin and heparinized saline irrigation, there is less agreement on pharmacologic regimens to improve anastomotic success in MFTT. Arterial vasospasm is a well-known complication that can lead to thrombosis, decreased flow, and ultimately flap failure. Papaverine, verapamil, and lidocaine are vasodilators that can be administered topically and are frequently utilized to minimize vasospasm.[34] In univariate and multivariate analyses, the local application of papaverine improved the success rate of vascular anastomosis.[3] However, there is no universal agreement on which, or how many, anti-spasmodic agent(s) should be used.

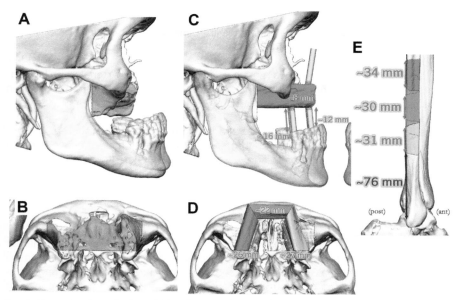

Fig. 1. Example of medical modeling for complex maxillary reconstruction. Sagittal and axial views with red-shaded area demonstrating bony resection (*A, B*). Sagittal and axial view of 3-segment fibular free flap to be used in reconstruction (*C, D*). Yellow columns projecting inferiorly represent dental implants. Yellow column projecting superiorly represents support post for a facial prosthetic as the patient had previously undergone total rhinectomy. Panel (*E*) demonstrates planned osteotomies and segments in the fibula.

Similarly, while some literature has suggested that intraoperative vasopressor use may compromise flap viability, more recent data has shown that vasopressor use has no bearing on anastomotic flow.[35] At the authors' institution, the authors routinely use topical lidocaine and variably papaverine. Practice regarding vasopressor use is varied, but, when necessary, the authors prefer low-dose phenylephrine infusion rather than bolus. As per ERAS protocols, the authors avoid over-transfusion of crystalloid product and encourage blood transfusion when needed.

Tranexamic Acid Use

Head and neck reconstructive surgery is inherently a procedure with long duration and thus variable blood loss. The presence of a pedicle in the neck can cause hematoma occurrence to be devastating for a patient's airway or free flap. To reduce hematoma rates and blood loss, tranexamic acid (TXA) has been studied across many surgical subspecialties. In patients undergoing head and neck surgery, TXA was found to significantly reduce intraoperative bleeding rates in patients undergoing tonsillectomy. Additionally, a randomized double-blinded, controlled study of preoperative TXA in 84 patients undergoing head and neck surgery showed TXA reduced blood loss and the need for transfusion as compared to placebo.[36] In another study, postoperative drain volumes were significantly reduced in patients undergoing major head and neck surgeries who received TXA.[37,38] While data remain inconclusive across surgical specialties, TXA does seem to be a safe and feasible medication to trial in head and neck patients who undergo MFTT and are at high risk for hematoma formation.[39]

Coupler Devices

First invented in 1962, and widely adopted in 1986, venous couplers have significantly reduced operative time and have been demonstrated to be safe, easy to use, and maintain vessel patency.[40] While venous coupler devices are now widely used, arterial anastomotic devices remain under development. Arterial coupling represents additional challenges, including a thicker wall to penetrate with the coupling device, and greater flow necessitating increased strength of the coupling system. Additionally, coupling may not be possible in severely atherosclerotic vessels. Nonetheless, arterial coupling can be a helpful adjunct in select cases, such as in scenarios when arterial anastomosis has thrombosed numerous times.[41] Vascular flow analysis of coupled anastomoses suggests that the coupler device may result in higher velocity laminar flow.[41] To address the challenges of arterial coupling with existing devices, new arterial couplers with a sheathing style mechanism are under development.[42]

Exoscope Technology

Magnification, whether through loupes or the use of a microscope, is essential for microvascular anastomosis. Recently introduced, exoscopes may offer an alternative for magnification. Using a 3-D camera placed above the surgical field, the magnification and visualization can be controlled by the surgeon but does not require looking through a lens. Advantages to exoscope technology include greater surgical operating view with uniform visualization for all, improved ergonomics, and greater teaching opportunities. Prior literature notes that exoscope use in head and neck microvascular surgery had similar operative times, anastomotic times, and free flap survival compared to operative microscopy use across 50 reconstructive patients.[43] While not widely used, exoscopes may also soon be used during ablation.

POSTOPERATIVE

Postoperative care for head and neck cancer patients undergoing MFTT has largely focused on optimizing MFTT outcomes while improving patient care and reducing hospital costs.

Free Flap Monitoring

Free flap monitoring remains an essential part of postoperative care. Many institutions rely on nursing staff to perform frequent (q1-2 hours) assessments of the flap color and Doppler sonography during the postoperative course. Some recent literature highlights that frequency of resident flap checks (eg,: every 4h vs every 12 h) does not alter free flap viability.[44] Further, implantable Dopplers are a commonly used probe that can be attached to the arterial pedicle to allow for real-time, continuous monitoring. Implantable Dopplers are particularly helpful in situations where no external cutaneous paddle is available for clinical monitoring.

New technology such as near-infrared spectroscopy (NIRS) is a postoperative adjunct used to measure tissue perfusion. Tissue perfusion is measured by detecting the percentage of oxygen-bound hemoglobin, which is a marker for tissue oxygen consumption and tissue health.[45] Proponents believe it provides a global view of the tissue compared to assessing pedicle perfusion alone. NIRS is routinely used in breast reconstruction with significant improvement in early detection of and overall flap salvage rates, but is less frequently utilized in head and neck reconstruction, due to inconvenient (eg,: intraoral) location of skin paddle. Nonetheless, this technology may offer superior monitoring in patients with large cutaneous reconstructions.

Improving Hospital Efficiency

As free flap volumes have increased substantially, hospital systems have sought to improve efficiency in postoperative care. At many institutions (including the authors' own), patients are not admitted to the intensive care unit (ICU) for postoperative care but rather an intermediate level head and neck floor, where nursing staff are familiar with head and neck patients and free flap reconstruction. Patients admitted to a step-down or general floor care had slightly higher flap success rate than those admitted to the ICU (97.0% vs 95.3%, $P = .02$).[46] While not logistically possible at all institutions, further benefits of this transition include decreased hospital costs, reduced nursing and staff handoffs, and postoperative patient care management by the surgical team primarily.[47,48]

Managing Donor-Site Morbidity

Many patients undergo full-thickness or split thickness skin grafts for coverage of donor site wounds. To encourage skin graft take, various techniques have been used, including long-term bolsters, wound vacuum negative pressure devices, or delayed skin grafting using synthetic dermal regeneration templates. Many of these options yield similar outcomes and are a matter of hospital resources and surgeon preference.[49] Although dermal regeneration substances generally require a 2-stage surgical approach, previous literature has highlighted potentially improved functionality and cosmesis with this approach.[50,51]

Dental Restoration

Tumors of the head and neck often require mandibular or maxillary resection, leaving patients edentulous. Osseointegrated dental implants can be performed at the time of (see earlier) or after reconstruction. Dental implants must be carefully chosen for the appropriate patient as they are not always anatomically possible or favorable, particularly in patients who have been irradiated.[52] A meta-analysis that investigated timing of dental implant placements found a slightly higher survival rate for the immediately placed dental implants, although there was no significant difference between the 2 groups.[53] In those whom dental implantation was successful, the investigators noted implant functionality ranged between 67.5% and 90.8%, although understanding true functional success can be challenging in this cohort.[53] Nonetheless, motivated and surgically appropriate patients for osseointegrated implants can have successful dental rehabilitation with the appropriate multidisciplinary surgical team.

Need for Salvage Surgery

Despite significant improvements in reconstruction, free flap failure and salvage surgery remains a frustrating component of microvascular surgery. Causes include pedicle compression from tissue edema or fluid collections, hypothyroidism, vessel thrombosis, and poorly controlled medical comorbidities. Swift return to the operating room to minimize ischemia time is essential for ultimate free flap survival.

Prior literature has evaluated patients necessitating 2 salvage reconstructive attempts, finding only 30% of doubly salvaged flaps survived. In those free flaps that did survive, arterial clots with subsequent revision led to a greater chance of success compared to those without an isolated pathology.[54] Notably, intravenous heparin is commonly used in cases of free flap failure; this study did not demonstrate increased free flap survival with the use of intravenous heparin. While these data are not favorable, it may be a helpful guide to surgeons in the setting of multiple threatened free flaps in the same patient and expected outcomes.

FUTURE DIRECTIONS
Bioresorbable Reconstruction

Current materials used in implantable plates generally include inert metals such as titanium. Titanium plates are often palpable, can seed infection, and sometimes require removal. However, ongoing research is investigating the use of biomaterials that resorb, ultimately leaving only native tissue remaining. Biomaterials used for surgical reconstruction have been previously used in partial airway reconstruction and in orthognathic surgery.[55,56] While nascent, maxillary and mandibular reconstruction using bioresorbable materials holds promise for head and neck reconstruction and may improve postoperative functional outcomes in this patient population. However, it is unclear how these bioresorbable materials will respond to radiation or recurrence.

Tissue Engineering

Stem cell and tissue engineering may obviate the need for autologous free tissue. Tissue engineering aims to regenerate native tissue; to do so, it requires a cellular source, scaffold material, and exogenous growth factors.[57] Combined, these components theoretically allow for the regeneration of the host tissue. Previously, adipose-derived stem cells were shown to improve the viability of non-vascularized bone grafts with significant regeneration.[58] However, much of this research remains in in vitro phases, and processing can be prohibitively costly. Nonetheless, future directions that can allow for cell regeneration may allow significant advancements in head and neck reconstructive patients.

DISCLOSURES

The authors have no disclosures to report.

REFERENCES

1. Corbitt C, Skoracki RJ, Yu P, et al. Free flap failure in head and neck reconstruction. Head Neck 2014;36(10):1440–5.
2. Eskander A, Kang S, Tweel B, et al. Predictors of complications in patients receiving head and neck free flap reconstructive procedures. Otolaryngol neck Surg Off J Am Acad Otolaryngol Neck Surg 2018;158(5):839–47.
3. Lin Y, He JF, Zhang X, et al. Intraoperative factors associated with free flap failure in the head and neck region: a four-year retrospective study of 216 patients and review of the literature. Int J Oral Maxillofac Surg 2019;48(4):447–51.
4. Vos JD, Burkey BB. Functional outcomes after free flap reconstruction of the upper aerodigestive tract. Curr Opin Otolaryngol Head Neck Surg 2004;12(4). Available at: https://journals.lww.com/co-otolaryngology/fulltext/2004/08000/functional_outcomes_after_free_flap_reconstruction.7.aspx.
5. Fancy T, Huang AT, Kass JI, et al. Complications, mortality, and functional decline in patients 80 years or older undergoing major head and neck ablation and reconstruction. JAMA Otolaryngol Neck Surg 2019;145(12):1150–7.
6. Beausang ES, Ang EE, Lipa JE, et al. Microvascular free tissue transfer in elderly patients: The Toronto experience. Head Neck 2003;25(7):549–53.
7. Otsuki N, Furukawa T, Avinçsal MO, et al. Results of free flap reconstruction for patients aged 80 years or older with head and neck cancer. Auris Nasus Larynx 2020;47(1):123–7.
8. Dort JC, Farwell DG, Findlay M, et al. Optimal perioperative care in major head and neck cancer surgery with free flap reconstruction: a consensus review and

recommendations from the enhanced recovery after surgery society. JAMA Oto-laryngol Neck Surg 2017;143(3):292–303.

9. Moore J, Scoggins CR, Philips P, et al. Implementation of prehabilitation for major abdominal surgery and head and neck surgery: a simplified seven-day protocol. J Gastrointest Surg 2021;25(8):2076–82.

10. Treanor C, Kyaw T, Donnelly M. An international review and meta-analysis of pre-habilitation compared to usual care for cancer patients. J Cancer Surviv 2018; 12(1):64–73.

11. Kristensen MB, Isenring E, Brown B. Nutrition and swallowing therapy strategies for patients with head and neck cancer. Nutrition 2020;69:110548.

12. Rieke K, Schmid KK, Lydiatt W, et al. Depression and survival in head and neck cancer patients. Oral Oncol 2017;65:76–82.

13. Chen J, Dennis SK, Abouyared M. Sarcopenia and microvascular free flap recon-struction. Curr Opin Otolaryngol Head Neck Surg 2021;29(5). Available at: https://journals.lww.com/co-otolaryngology/fulltext/2021/10000/sarcopenia_and_microvascular_free_flap.13.aspx.

14. Mueller SA, Mayer C, Bojaxhiu B, et al. Effect of preoperative immunonutrition on complications after salvage surgery in head and neck cancer. J Otolaryngol - Head Neck Surg 2019;48(1).

15. Meuli JN, Guiotto M, Elmers J, et al. Outcomes after microsurgical treatment of lymphedema: a systematic review and meta-analysis. Int J Surg 2023;109(5). Available at: https://journals.lww.com/international-journal-of-surgery/fulltext/2023/05000/outcomes_after_microsurgical_treatment_of.32.aspx.

16. Mihara M, Uchida G, Hara H, et al. Lymphaticovenous anastomosis for facial lym-phoedema after multiple courses of therapy for head-and-neck cancer. J Plast Reconstr Aesthetic Surg 2011;64(9):1221–5.

17. Farlow JL, McCrary HC, Li M, et al. Internal jugular vein reconstruction: An algo-rithm for reconstructive surgeons. Oral Oncol 2023;145:106523.

18. Agarwal R, Freeman TE, Li MM, et al. Outcomes with culture-directed antibiotics following microvascular free tissue reconstruction for osteonecrosis of the jaw. Oral Oncol 2022;130:105878.

19. Jacobson AS, Eloy JA, Park E, et al. Vessel-depleted neck: Techniques for achieving microvascular reconstruction. Head Neck 2008;30(2):201–7.

20. Chen Y-W, Yen J-H, Chen W-H, et al. Preoperative computed tomography angiog-raphy for evaluation of feasibility of free flaps in difficult reconstruction of head and neck. Ann Plast Surg 2016;76. Available at: https://journals.lww.com/annalsplasticsurgery/fulltext/2016/03001/preoperative_computed_tomography_angiography_for.4.aspx.

21. Urken ML, Higgins KM, Lee B, et al. Internal mammary artery and vein: Recipient vessels for free tissue transfer to the head and neck in the vessel-depleted neck. Head Neck 2006;28(9):797–801.

22. Prince ADP, Broderick MT, Heft Neal ME, et al. Head and neck reconstruction in the vessel depleted neck. Front Oral Maxillofac Med 2020;2.

23. Martinez DC, Badhey A, Cervenka B, et al. Surgical techniques for head and neck reconstruction in the vessel-depleted neck. Facial Plast Surg 2020;36(6): 746–52.

24. Seim NB, Old M, Petrisor D, et al. Head and neck free flap survival when requiring interposition vein grafting: A multi-instiutional review. Oral Oncol 2020;101: 104482.

25. Langdell HC, Shammas RL, Atia A, et al. Vein grafts in free flap reconstruction: review of indications and institutional pearls. Plast Reconstr Surg 2022;149(3): 742–9.

26. Annino DJ, Hansen EE, Sethi RK, et al. Accuracy and outcomes of virtual surgical planning and 3D-printed guides for osseous free flap reconstruction of mandibular osteoradionecrosis. Oral Oncol 2022;135.

27. Seim NB, Ozer E, Valentin S, et al. Custom presurgical planning for midfacial reconstruction. Facial Plast Surg 2020;36(6):696–702.

28. McCrary HC, Seim NB, Old MO. History, innovation, pearls, and pitfalls in complex midface reconstruction. Otolaryngol Clin North Am 2023;56(4):703–13.

29. Nyirjesy SC, Heller M, von Windheim N, et al. The role of computer aided design/ computer assisted manufacturing (CAD/CAM) and 3- dimensional printing in head and neck oncologic surgery: A review and future directions. Oral Oncol 2022;132.

30. Moore EJ, Price DL, Van Abel KM, et al. Association of virtual surgical planning with external incisions in complex maxillectomy reconstruction. JAMA Otolaryngol Neck Surg 2021;147(6):526–31.

31. Qaisi M, Zheng W, Al Azzawi T, et al. Patient specific bony and soft-tissue fibular reconstruction: Perforator virtual surgical planning technique. Adv Oral Maxillofac Surg 2022;8:100363.

32. Chen SY, Lin WC, Deng SC, et al. Assessment of the perforators of anterolateral thigh flaps using 64-section multidetector computed tomographic angiography in head and neck cancer reconstruction. Eur J Surg Oncol J Eur Soc Surg Oncol Br Assoc Surg Oncol 2010;36(10):1004–11.

33. Eskander A, Kang SY, Teknos TN, et al. Advances in midface reconstruction: Beyond the reconstructive ladder. Curr Opin Otolaryngol Head Neck Surg 2017;25(5):422–30.

34. Yu JTS, Patel AJK, Malata CM. The use of topical vasodilators in microvascular surgery. J Plast Reconstr Aesthetic Surg 2011;64(2):226–8.

35. Naik AN, Freeman T, Li MM, et al. The use of vasopressor agents in free tissue transfer for head and neck reconstruction: current trends and review of the literature. Front Pharmacol 2020;11(August).

36. Babu MJ, Neema PK, Reazaul Karim HM, et al. Effect of two different tranexamic acid doses on blood loss in head and neck cancer surgery: a randomized, double-blind, controlled study. Cureus 2021;13(12).

37. Jamshaid W, Jamshaid M, Coulson C, et al. A systematic review on the efficacy of tranexamic acid in head and neck surgery. Clin Otolaryngol 2023;48(4):527–39.

38. Yan Z, Chen S, Xue T, et al. The function of tranexamic acid to prevent hematoma expansion after intracerebral hemorrhage: a systematic review and meta-analysis from randomized controlled trials. Front Neurol 2021;12.

39. Klifto KM, Hanwright PJ, Sacks JM. Tranexamic acid in microvascular free flap reconstruction. Plast Reconstr Surg 2020;146(4):517E–8E.

40. Frederick JW, Sweeny L, Carroll WR, et al. Microvascular anastomotic coupler assessment in head and neck reconstruction. Otolaryngol neck Surg Off J Am Acad Otolaryngol Neck Surg 2013;149(1):67–70.

41. Li MM, Tamaki A, Seim NB, et al. Utilization of microvascular couplers in salvage arterial anastomosis in head and neck free flap surgery: Case series and literature review. Head Neck 2020;42(8):E1–7.

42. Jeong W, Kim K, Son D, et al. New Absorbable Microvascular Anastomotic Devices Representing a Modified Sleeve Technique: Evaluation of Two Types of Source Material and Design. Sci Rep 2019;9(1):10945.

43. De Virgilio A, Costantino A, Russo E, et al. Comparison between the high-definition 3D exoscope and the operating microscope in head and neck reconstruction. Int J Oral Maxillofac Surg 2023.
44. Patel UA, Hernandez D, Shnayder Y, et al. Free flap reconstruction monitoring techniques and frequency in the era of restricted resident work hours. JAMA Otolaryngol Head Neck Surg 2017;143(8):803–9.
45. Starr NC, Slade E, Gal TJ, et al. Remote monitoring of head and neck free flaps using near infrared spectroscopic tissue oximetry. Am J Otolaryngol - Head Neck Med Surg 2021;42(1).
46. Kovatch KJ, Hanks JE, Stevens JR, et al. Current practices in microvascular reconstruction in otolaryngology–head and neck surgery. Laryngoscope 2019; 129(1):138–45.
47. Varadarajan VV, Arshad H, Dziegielewski PT. Head and neck free flap reconstruction: What is the appropriate post-operative level of care? Oral Oncol 2017; 75:61–6.
48. Arshad H, Ozer HG, Thatcher A, et al. Intensive care unit versus non–intensive care unit postoperative management of head and neck free flaps: Comparative effectiveness and cost comparisons. Head Neck 2014;36(4):536–9.
49. Halama D, Dreilich R, Lethaus B, et al. Donor-site morbidity after harvesting of radial forearm free flaps—comparison of vacuum-assisted closure with conventional wound care: A randomized controlled trial. J Cranio-Maxillofacial Surg 2019;47(12):1980–5.
50. Reece MK, Walker H, Benintendi I, et al. Delayed skin grafting protocol following Integra™ application for non-radiated scalp reconstruction for decreased wound depth and improved contour. Head Neck 2023;45(11):2967–74.
51. Murray RC, Gordin EA, Saigal K, et al. Reconstruction of the radial forearm free flap donor site using integra artificial dermis. Microsurgery 2011;31(2):104–8.
52. Lodders JN, Leusink FKJ, Ridwan-Pramana A, et al. Long-term outcomes of implant-based dental rehabilitation in head and neck cancer patients after reconstruction with the free vascularized fibula flap. J Cranio-Maxillofacial Surg 2021; 49(9):845–54.
53. in 't Veld M, Schulten EAJM, Leusink FKJ. Immediate dental implant placement and restoration in the edentulous mandible in head and neck cancer patients: a systematic review and meta-analysis. Curr Opin Otolaryngol Head Neck Surg. 2021;29(2). Available at: https://journals.lww.com/co-otolaryngology/fulltext/2021/04000/immediate_dental_implant_placement_and_restoration.10.aspx.
54. Slijepcevic AA, Young G, Shinn J, et al. Success and Outcomes Following a Second Salvage Attempt for Free Flap Compromise in Patients Undergoing Head and Neck Reconstruction. JAMA Otolaryngol Head Neck Surg 2022;148(6): 555–60.
55. Les AS, Ohye RG, Filbrun AG, et al. 3D-printed, externally-implanted, bioresorbable airway splints for severe tracheobronchomalacia. Laryngoscope 2019;129(8):1763–71.
56. Kanno T, Sukegawa S, Furuki Y, et al. Overview of innovative advances in bioresorbable plate systems for oral and maxillofacial surgery. Jpn Dent Sci Rev 2018;54(3):127–38.
57. Shaul JL, Davis BK, Burg KJL. Regenerative Engineering in Maxillofacial Reconstruction. Regen Eng Transl Med 2016;2(2):55–68.
58. Lendeckel S, Jödicke A, Christophis P, et al. Autologous stem cells (adipose) and fibrin glue used to treat widespread traumatic calvarial defects: Case report. J Cranio-Maxillofacial Surg 2004;32(6):370–3.

Updates in the Management of Advanced Nonmelanoma Skin Cancer

Flora Yan, MD, Cecelia E. Schmalbach, MD, MSc*

KEYWORDS

- Nonmelanoma skin cancer • Basal cell carcinoma
- Cutaneous squamous cell carcinoma • Merkel cell carcinoma
- Cutaneous malignancies

KEY POINTS

- Nonmelanoma skin cancer (NMSC), mainly comprised of basal cell carcinoma (BCC), cutaneous squamous cell carcinoma (cSCC), and Merkel cell carcinoma (MCC), is increasing at epidemic rates due to our aging patient population, environmental changes, successful organ transplantation, and sun-worshiping behaviors.
- BCC and cSCC of the head and neck region are automatically classified as high-risk lesions.
- MCC of any location is considered an aggressive and high-risk entity.
- Systemic therapy options for NMSC are expanding. Hedgehog inhibitors (HHIs) have become integral in the management of recurrent/metastatic BCC.
- Immune checkpoint inhibitors have a significant role for BCC patients who fail HHIs as well as for recurrent and metastatic cSCC and MCC patients failing traditional therapy.

INTRODUCTION

Nonmelanoma skin cancer (NMSC) is a heterogeneous category of cutaneous cancers, with basal cell carcinoma (BCC), cutaneous squamous cell carcinoma (cSCC), and Merkel cell carcinoma (MCC) accounting for the vast majority. The incidence of NMSC is increasing likely due to our aging population, successful organ transplantation, sun-worshiping behaviors, and changing environmental factors. Using data from the Global Burden of Disease 2019 study, Hu and colleagues[1] demonstrated an increase in the age-standardized incidence rate from 54.08/100,000 in 1990 to 79.10/100,000 in 2019.[2,3] The ever-growing global incidence underscores the importance of continual advances in the management of NMSC.

Department of Otolaryngology–Head & Neck Surgery, Lewis Katz School of Medicine at Temple Hospital, Philadelphia, PA, USA
* Corresponding author. 3440 North Broad Street Kresge West #300, Philadelphia, PA 19140.
E-mail address: cecelia.schmalbach@tuhs.temple.edu

Surg Oncol Clin N Am 33 (2024) 723–733
https://doi.org/10.1016/j.soc.2024.04.006
1055-3207/24/© 2024 Elsevier Inc. All rights reserved.
surgonc.theclinics.com

BCC is the most common skin cancer worldwide, accounting for 75% to 80% of all NMSCs with 80% occurring in the head and neck region.[4],[5] Nodular BCC accounts for the most common variant (60%–80%) and presents as a nodular or popular pearly lesion.[6] Superficial BCCs are the second most common variant (20%), present as a scaly, pink macule[5],[6] with a tendency to regress. Morpheaform/sclerosing BCC is a higher risk subtype that presents as a pink and ivory-colored plaque with telangiectasias and ulcerations. This variant has a higher rate of recurrence and perineural invasion (PNI) than nodular or superficial BCCs.[7–9] Overall, BCC have a very low rate of metastasis at 0.0028% to 0.5%;[10],[11] however, at times, BCC can locally invade tissues, resulting in high morbidity following resection. Higher risk subtypes as well as the presence of pathologic risk factors such as PNI increase rates of recurrence (**Table 1**).

cSCC is the second most common NMSC, accounting for 20% to 25% of NMSCs.[12] The overall risk of recurrence is 5%, with a 4% to 6% risk of nodal and distant metastases.[12] These cancers often appear as scaly, ulcerated nodules or plaques.[13]

BCCs and cSCCs share similar risk factors that include cumulative ultraviolet light exposure, advanced age, radiation therapy (RT), arsenic exposure, fair skin, and a history of immunosuppression. Patients with Fitzpatrick skin types I and II have a 30% lifetime risk of developing BCCs.[6] Immunosuppressed populations include human immunodeficiency virus (HIV)–positive patients and solid organ transplant (SOT) recipients carry a 2-fold and 5-fold increased incidence of BCC compared to their immunocompetent counterparts.[14] SOT recipients develop cSCC at even higher rates, with 65 to 250 times greater risk compared to the general population.[15],[16] Lastly, there are a host of genetic syndromes associated with BCC and SCC: xeroderma pigmentosa (BCC and SCC), epidermolysis bullosa (SCC), basal cell nevus syndrome/ Gorlin's syndrome (BCC), Rombo syndrome (BCC), and Bazex-Dupre-Christol syndrome (BCC).[12]

MCC is a rare and aggressive neuroendocrine tumor that presents as a rapidly growing, violaceous nodule which is often mistaken for BCC. Up to 26% of cases present with regional disease and an additional 8% present with distant metastases.[17–21] Five-year overall survival rates range from 48% to 63%.[17] The Merkel cell polyomavirus (MCP-yV) has been highly implicated in the pathogenesis of MCC, with integration of the MCP-yV within the genome of tumor cells, leading to malignant transformation as a mechanism of MCC development. Up to 80% of MCC tumors have been associated with the MCP-yV as evidenced by the genomic integration of the MCP-yV gene in cellular DNA.[22],[23] Importantly, virus-negative patients may represent a more aggressive subtype, with an increased risk of disease progression and death from MCC than that of virus-positive tumors.[24]

NONMELANOMA SKIN CANCER RISK STRATIFICATION

The National Comprehensive Cancer Network (NCCN) guidelines differentiate the risk of recurrence of NMSC by a variety of clinical and pathologic factors. BCC is divided into low and high risk, whereas cSCC is divided in low-risk, high-risk, and very high–risk lesions. **Table 1** summarizes the various factors utilized in risk stratification. In addition, the "H-zone of the face (ie, nasolabial fold, nasal ala, and orbital and periauricular regions) have higher rates of recurrence.[25] Size $\geq$ 2 cm on any other site (trunk and extremities) is considered high risk. Any history of malignancies, particularly SOT recipients, can increase the risk of aggressive disease. PNI is a rare occurrence in NMSC; however, if it occurs, it poses a high risk of recurrence and is usually found in conjunction with other high-risk features such as large lesion size and recurrent

Table 1
High-risk head and neck basal cell carcinoma[26] and cutaneous squamous cell carcinoma[41] features

Characteristics	High-Risk Basal Cell Carcinoma	High-Risk Cutaneous Squamous Cell Carcinoma	Very-High-Risk Cutaneous Squamous Cell Carcinoma
Size	≥ 2 cm of the trunk or extremities	2–4 cm on trunk or extremities	>4 cm
Depth/thickness	—	2–6 mm depth	>6 mm or invasion beyond subcutaneous fat
Borders	Poorly defined	Poorly defined	—
Histology	• Basosquamous • Infiltrative • Sclerosing/morpheaform • Micronodular • Carcinosarcomatous	• Acantholytic • Adenosquamous • Metaplastic	Desmoplastic
Grade	—	—	Poor differentiation
Pathologic features	Any PNI	PNI < 0.1 mm	• PNI ≥ 0.1 mm • Tumor within nerve sheath of nerve deeper than dermis • Any LVI
Symptoms	—	• Rapid growth • Neurologic symptoms	—
History	• Prior radiation therapy • Recurrent disease • Immunosuppression	• Prior radiation therapy • Recurrent disease • Immunosuppression	—

Abbreviations: LVI, lymphovascular invasion; PNI, perineural invasion.

disease.[26] It should be noted that all cSCCs and BCCs of the head and neck are automatically considered at least high risk regardless of size.

There is not a distinct risk stratification system for MCC; the NCCN does identify adverse risk factors that prompt additional multimodality treatment. These include primary tumor greater than 1 cm, chronic T-cell immunosuppression, HIV, chronic lymphocytic leukemia, SOT with head/neck as the primary site, and presence of lymphovascular invasion (LVI).[27]

ADVANCES IN BASAL CELL CARCINOMA TREATMENT

Surgical resection with a minimum of 6-mm margins remains the standard of care for high-risk tumors.[26] This can be achieved through wide local excision or Mohs micrographic surgery (MMS) which provides the advantage of a comprehensive 360-degree histopathological margin evaluation in a tissue-sparing manner. MMS is recommended for high-risk BCCs as well as those in cosmetically sensitive locations such as near the eyelids, nose, ears, or lips.[28,29] Primary RT is considered the first-line treatment for nonsurgical candidates.

The hedgehog signaling pathway is responsible for basal cell proliferation and subsequent tumor growth.[30] Hedgehog inhibitors (HHIs) remain the first-line treatment for recurrent, metastatic, or locally advanced BCC that is not responsive to surgery or radiation. There are currently 2 Food and Drug Administration (FDA)–approved HHI for BCC: vismodegib (2012) and sonidegib (2015). Both agents inhibit the cell surface receptor smoothened homolog, a key protein in the activation of the hedgehog signaling pathway.[31] The challenge is that the 30% to 40% of patients require a drug holiday secondary to arthralgias and other side effects.[32]

The optimal management of advanced BCC with HHIs continues to be refined. The BOLT (A Phase II Study of Efficacy and Safety in Patients With Locally Advanced or Metastatic Basal Cell Carcinoma) trial, evaluating sonidegib, demonstrated a 60% overall response rate (ORR),[33] whereas the ERIVANCE (A Study Evaluating the Efficacy and Safety of Vismodegib (GDC-0449, Hedgehog Pathway Inhibitor) in Patients With Advanced Basal Cell Carcinoma) trial, evaluating vismodegib, demonstrated a 47.6% response rate.[34] The optimal duration of HHI therapy remains to be determined; treatment usually continues until the patient experiences complete remission, treatment toxicity, or disease progression.[35] Additionally, HHIs in the advanced BCC neoadjuvant setting is an area of active study. Neoadjuvant HHIs may allow for downstaging of a tumor prior to surgical treatment and may decrease the morbidity of resection.[35] The VISMONEO (Study Evaluating the Interest of Vismodegib as Neo-adjuvant Treatment of Basal Cell Carcinoma) study, a multi-center phase 2 trial, evaluated vismodegib in the neoadjuvant study in patients with anatomically or cosmetically/functionally inoperable facial BCC and demonstrated a 71% ORR; 80% of patients were able to be downstaged after vismodegib treatment.[36]

Patients who fail surgery, radiation, and HHI therapy are candidates for immune checkpoint inhibitors (ICIs). Cemiplimab, a programmed cell death protein-1 (PD-1) inhibitor became FDA approved in 2021 for systemic treatment of advanced BCC patients in this setting. Data from a multicenter single-arm phase 2 trial evaluating cemiplimab therapy in patients with advanced BCC who had previously failed HHI therapy demonstrated a 31% overall objective response.[37] There has been evidence that HHIs can increase the immunogenicity of BCCs and allow for increased effectiveness of PD-1 inhibitors.[38,39] A potential treatment regimen could include HHI with PD-1 inhibitors in combination after failure on HHIs alone. Further studies would need to demonstrate efficacy of this prior to implementation.[35]

ADVANCES IN CUTANEOUS SQUAMOUS CELL CARCINOMA TREATMENT

For high-risk cSCC, the standard of care remains surgical resection with the goal of complete clearance of the cancer. The ideal surgical margin size remains a topic of active debate. Brodland and colleagues[40] performed a prospective study of subclinical microscopic tumor extension to evaluate tumor clearance after resection. They concluded that high-risk cSCCs require margins based on diameter: lesions less than 1 cm requiring at least 4-mm margins, lesions 1 to 1.9 cm requiring at least 6-mm margins, and lesions $\geq$ 2 cm requiring at least 9-mm gross margins in order to histologically clear all disease.[40] The current European guidelines recommend a 6-mm to 10-mm margin for high-risk and very-high-risk lesions.[37] Given the variability of characteristics used to define high risk and the differing prognostic implications, there has been no well-defined margin recommended by the NCCN.[41]

Patients with biopsy-proven regional disease warrant a therapeutic lymphadenectomy to address their N-positive neck. It is important to keep in mind that tumors arising on the high cheek, forehead, and temple region warrant a superficial parotidectomy in addition to addressing the cervical nodes. Tumors arising behind an imaginary coronal plane through the external auditory canal require a posterior lateral neck dissection to include the suboccipital and retroauricular nodes.

Management of the clinically node-negative (N0) neck is based on the risk of occult nodal metastasis. The rate of metastatic regional spread may be as high as 47% in the high-risk and very high-risk cSCC population, especially in the setting of tumor recurrence and immunosuppression.[42] For this reason, elective neck dissection of at risk nodal basins can be offered to patients. Alternatively, sentinel node biopsy (SLNB) provides an alternative option with minimal surgical morbidity. Meta-analysis of head and neck cSCC patients staged with SLNB demonstrated false omission rate of 4.76% which is comparable to melanoma where SLNB is considered the standard of care. In addition, several reports demonstrate improved locoregional and distant recurrence rates as well as improving disease-specific or overall survival in the setting of cSCC SLNB staging.[43–47] Currently the American Head & Neck Society recognizes cSCC SLNB as the most sensitive and specific staging modality for cSCC patients[48] and the NCCN encourages an SLNB discussion for very high-risk cSCC patient that are recurrent or have multiple risk factors as outlined earlier.[41]

Primary radiation is an acceptable alternative treatment option for patients with unresectable tumors or who are medically unfit for surgery. A meta-analysis including 14 observational studies examining primary RT for nonmetastatic cSCC demonstrated a mean local recurrence rate of 6.4%.[49–51] External beam RT is the most common modality and is either electron or proton based. Electron-based RT is used to treat superficial lesions whereas photon-based RT has greater penetrance and can be used for deeper lesions. Side effects of RT include acute dermatitis, late-onset depigmentation, and telangiectasias.[37] For this reason, primary RT is generally reserved for the elderly, as long-term side effects may be more pronounced with aging. RT can also be considered in the adjuvant setting. Adjuvant RT is indicated for patients with close surgical margins not amenable to re-resection, PNI, tumors $\geq$6 cm in diameter, recurrent tumors, high-risk histologic subtypes, or for patients who are chronically immunosuppressed.[41]

The advent of ICIs has changed the landscape for cSCC systemic treatment.[48] Currently, the first-line treatment for metastatic or locally advanced cSCC not amenable to surgery or RT is a PD-1 inhibitor (**Table 2**).[41,52] Currently there are 2 FDA-approved ICIs for cSCC: cemiplimab (2018) and pembrolizumab (2020). The EMPOWER-CSCC-1 (Study of REGN2810 in Patients With Advanced Cutaneous

Table 2
Indications for programmed cell death protein-1 inhibitor immunotherapy for cutaneous squamous cell carcinoma

Patient factors	Comorbidities precluding surgery
	Surgery would result in severe disfigurement/dysfunction
	Patient preference to avoid surgery or radiation therapy
	Unresectable disease (ie, skull base; carotid)
Treatment factors	Failed curative intent surgery or radiation therapy

Squamous Cell Carcinoma) trial, a phase II multicenter trial, demonstrated a 47% ORR using cemiplimab in patients with metastatic or locally advanced cSCC.[53] Additionally, the KEYNOTE-629 (Study of Pembrolizumab (MK-3475) in Adults With Recurrent/Metastatic Cutaneous Squamous Cell Carcinoma (cSCC) or Locally Advanced Unresectable cSCC) trial, a phase II multicenter single arm trial, investigated the efficacy of pembrolizumab and demonstrated a 50% and 35% ORR for patient with metastatic and locally advanced cSCC, respectively.[54] It is important to note that these trials exclude SOT patients or those with hematological malignancies due to the high rejection rate.[52] Cemiplimab has also been examined in the neoadjuvant setting. In a pilot study with 79 stage II, III, and IV cSCC patients receiving neoadjuvant cemiplimab followed by curative intent surgery, it was demonstrated a pathologic complete response in 51% and a pathologic major response rate (<10% remaining tumor) in an additional 13% of patients. Further studies aim to delineate the role of cemiplimab in the neoadjuvant setting.[55] For patients who are immunosuppressed and those who failed immune checkpoint inhibition or could not tolerate it, cetuximab, an epidermal growth factor receptor (EGFR) inhibitor, can be used as monotherapy or in combination with RT.[37,41]

Previously, systemic platinum-based chemotherapy options were considered for cSCC including cisplatin and carboplatin. The consideration of platinum-based therapies was initially proposed given the efficacy of these agents in mucosal head and neck SCC. The TROG 05.01 (Post-operative Concurrent Chemo-radiotherapy Versus Post-operative Radiotherapy for Cancer of the Head and Neck) trial investigated postoperative RT versus postoperative chemoradiation therapy in patients with high-risk cSCC and demonstrated both treatment regimens exhibiting comparable regional recurrence rates; however, no overt survival improvements were seen with the addition of carboplatin.[56] The authors note limitations to the study including lack of power to detect smaller benefits from chemotherapy and the use of carboplatin rather than cisplatin.[56] Currently, the use of platinum-based chemotherapy is reserved for patients who fail of immune checkpoint or EGFR-inhibition.[37]

ADVANCES IN MERKEL CELL CARCINOMA TREATMENT

Similar to BCC and cSCC, the first-line treatment for MCC is surgical resection. The NCCN guidelines recommend 1-cm to 2-cm gross margins, with potential for narrower margins if postoperative RT was planned.[27] This recommendation was largely based on a review of data from the national cancer database that examined the association of surgical margin status in patients with MCC.[57] Adjuvant RT should be considered for most cases of MCC, especially those with adverse risk factors such as tumor size greater than 1 cm, LVI, head and neck as the primary site, or immunosuppression.[27,58]

SLNB is the standard of care for N0 MCC patients because up to one-third of cases of MCC harbor occult nodal metastases.[59] In this setting, it is used as a staging modality. Evidence suggests that positive SLNB is associated with decreased overall and disease specific survival, acting as a key prognosticator for MCC.[60,61] However, the true impact of SLNB on MCC recurrence and survival is unclear with conflicting literature and it remains an area of study.[62–64]

Similar to cSCC, systemic therapy options for MCC largely stem around ICIs. To date, there are 3 FDA-approved immunotherapy options for MCC: avelumab (anti-programmed death-ligand 1 inhibitor), pembrolizumab, and most recently, retifanlimab-dlwr (anti-PD-1 inhibitor).[65] Avelumab was approved for use in MCC in 2017 after results from the JAVELIN Merkel 200 (Avelumab in Participants With Merkel Cell Carcinoma) trial demonstrated an ORR of 32%.[66] Additionally, results from a global expanded access program evaluating real-world experiences of patients with MCC treated with avelumab demonstrated an ORR of 47%.[67] Pembrolizumab was approved in 2018 based on data from the KEYNOTE-017 (Pembrolizumab in Treating Patients With Advanced Merkel Cell Cancer) trial which demonstrated an ORR of 56%.[68] Retinfanlimab-dlwr was recently FDA approved in 2023 after results of PODIUM-201 (A Study of INCMGA00012 in Metastatic Merkel Cell Carcinoma), an open-label, multiregional, single-arm study, demonstrated an ORR of 52% in patients with metastatic or recurrent locally advanced MCC.[69] Current investigations are ongoing to evaluate the role of nivolumab in the neoadjuvant and adjuvant settings for MCC.[70,71] The phase I/II CheckMate 358 (An Investigational Immuno-therapy Study to Investigate the Safety and Effectiveness of Nivolumab, and Nivolumab Combination Therapy in Virus-associated Tumors) trial demonstrated that neoadjuvant nivolumab in patients with MCC was tolerable and also effective. Of 39 patients enrolled with resectable MCC who received nivolumab 4 weeks prior to surgery, 47% achieved a pathologic complete response.[70]

SUMMARY

NMSC is growing in incidence at epidemic proportions. High-risk features of NMSC are being investigated to delineate specific prognostic impact. Systemic treatment options for all NMSCs are expanded with the advent of ICIs. Areas of future study include the role of SLNB for cSCC, the potential use of PD-1 inhibitors in immunosuppressed populations with cSCC, and treatment strategies for patients refractory to ICIs and HHIs.

CLinics CARE POINTS

- The incidence of NMSC is growing at epidemic proportions.
- High-rish features of NMSC are being investigated to delineate specific prognostic impact; at a minimum all BCC and cSCC diagnosed in the Head & Neck region are considered high risk.
- SLNBx is considered standard of care for node negative cSCC and MCC harboring high risk of occult metastasis.
- Systemic therapy is reserved for recalcitrant NMSCs refractory to surgery and/or radiation.
- Hedge Hog inhibitors remain first line for BCC systemic treatment, with immunotherapy being reserved for failures or ineligible patients.
- Immunotherapy (PD 1 inhibitors) are now approved for BCC, cSCC and MCC.

DISCLOSURE

None to disclose.

REFERENCES

1. Hu W, Fang L, Ni R, et al. Changing trends in the disease burden of non-melanoma skin cancer globally from 1990 to 2019 and its predicted level in 25 years. BMC Cancer 2022;22(1):836.
2. Staples MP, Elwood M, Burton RC, et al. Non-melanoma skin cancer in Australia: the 2002 national survey and trends since 1985. Med J Aust 2006;184(1):6–10.
3. Xiang F, Lucas R, Hales S, et al. Incidence of nonmelanoma skin cancer in relation to ambient UV radiation in white populations, 1978-2012: Empirical Relationships. JAMA Dermatology 2014;150(10):1063–71.
4. Samarasinghe V, Madan V. Nonmelanoma skin cancer. J Cutan Aesthet Surg 2012;5(1):3–10.
5. Scrivener Y, Grosshans E, Cribier B. Variations of basal cell carcinomas according to gender, age, location and histopathological subtype. Br J Dermatol 2002;147(1):41–7.
6. Naik PP, Desai MB. Basal cell carcinoma: a narrative review on contemporary diagnosis and management. Oncol Ther 2022;10(2):317–35.
7. Connolly AHTFSM, Baker DR, Coldiron BM, et al. AAD/ACMS/ASDSA/ASMS 2012 Appropriate Use Criteria for Mohs Micrographic Surgery: A Report of the A merican A cademy of D ermatology, American College of Mohs Surgery, American Society for Dermatologic S urgery Association, and the American Society for Mohs Surgery. Dermatol Surg 2012;38(10):1582–603.
8. Hendrix JD, Parlette HL. Micronodular basal cell carcinoma: a deceptive histologic subtype with frequent clinically undetected tumor extension. Arch Dermatol 1996;132(3):295–8.
9. Akay BN, Saral S, Heper AO, et al. Basosquamous carcinoma: dermoscopic clues to diagnosis. J Dermatol 2017;44(2):127–34.
10. Malone JP, Fedok FG, Belchis DA, et al. Basal cell carcinoma metastatic to the parotid: report of a new case and review of the literature. Ear Nose Throat J 2000;79(7):511–5, 518-519.
11. von Domarus H, Stevens PJ. Metastatic basal cell carcinoma. Report of five cases and review of 170 cases in the literature. J Am Acad Dermatol 1984;10(6):1043–60.
12. Cives M, Mannavola F, Lospalluti L, et al. Non-melanoma skin cancers: biological and clinical features. Int J Mol Sci 2020;21(15).
13. Fania L, Didona D, Morese R, et al. Basal cell carcinoma: from pathophysiology to novel therapeutic approaches. Biomedicines 2020;8(11):449.
14. Silverberg MJ, Leyden W, Warton EM, et al. HIV infection status, immunodeficiency, and the incidence of non-melanoma skin cancer. J Natl Cancer Inst 2013;105(5):350–60.
15. Greenberg JN, Zwald FO. Management of skin cancer in solid-organ transplant recipients: a multidisciplinary approach. Dermatol Clin 2011;29(2):231, 241, ix.
16. Moloney FJ, Comber H, O'Lorcain P, et al. A population-based study of skin cancer incidence and prevalence in renal transplant recipients. Br J Dermatol 2006; 154(3):498–504.
17. Gauci M-L, Aristei C, Becker JC, et al. Diagnosis and treatment of Merkel cell carcinoma: European consensus-based interdisciplinary guideline – Update 2022. Eur J Cancer 2022;171:203–31.
18. Toker C. Trabecular carcinoma of the skin. Arch Dermatol 1972;105(1):107–10.
19. Lemasson G, Coquart N, Lebonvallet N, et al. Presence of putative stem cells in Merkel cell carcinomas. J Eur Acad Dermatol Venereol 2012;26(6):789–95.

20. Visscher D, Cooper PH, Zarbo RJ, et al. Cutaneous neuroendocrine (Merkel cell) carcinoma: an immunophenotypic, clinicopathologic, and flow cytometric study. Mod Pathol 1989;2(4):331–8.
21. Zur Hausen A, Rennspiess D, Winnepenninckx V, et al. Early B-cell differentiation in Merkel cell carcinomas: clues to cellular ancestry. Cancer Res 2013;73(16):4982–7.
22. Feng H, Shuda M, Chang Y, et al. Clonal integration of a polyomavirus in human Merkel cell carcinoma. Science 2008;319(5866):1096–100.
23. Santos-Juanes J, Fernández-Vega I, Fuentes N, et al. Merkel cell carcinoma and Merkel cell polyomavirus: a systematic review and meta-analysis. Br J Dermatol 2015;173(1):42–9.
24. Moshiri AS, Doumani R, Yelistratova L, et al. Polyomavirus-negative merkel cell carcinoma: a more aggressive subtype based on analysis of 282 cases using multimodal tumor virus detection. J Invest Dermatol 2017;137(4):819–27.
25. Swanson NA, Grekin RC, Baker SR. Mohs surgery: techniques, indications, and applications in head and neck surgery. Head Neck Surg 1983;6(2):683–92.
26. National Comprehensive Cancer Network, Basal Cell Skin Cancer Version 3.2024, Available at: https://www.nccn.org/professionals/physician_gls/pdf/nmsc.pdf. (Accessed 27 May 2024), 2024.
27. National Comprehensive Cancer Network. Merkel Cell Carcinoma Version 1.2023. 2023. Available at: https://www.nccn.org/professionals/physician_gls/pdf/mcc.pdf. [Accessed 27 September 2023].
28. Connolly SM, Baker DR, Coldiron BM, et al. AAD/ACMS/ASDSA/ASMS 2012 appropriate use criteria for Mohs micrographic surgery: a report of the American Academy of Dermatology, American College of Mohs Surgery, American Society for Dermatologic Surgery Association, and the American Society for Mohs Surgery. J Am Acad Dermatol 2012;67(4):531–50.
29. Kauvar AN, Cronin T Jr, Roenigk R, et al. Consensus for nonmelanoma skin cancer treatment: basal cell carcinoma, including a cost analysis of treatment methods. Dermatol Surg 2015;41(5):550–71.
30. Epstein EH. Basal cell carcinomas: attack of the hedgehog. Nat Rev Cancer 2008;8(10):743–54.
31. Nguyen NM, Cho J. Hedgehog pathway inhibitors as targeted cancer therapy and strategies to overcome drug resistance. Int J Mol Sci 2022;23(3).
32. Sekulic A, Migden MR, Oro AE, et al. Efficacy and safety of vismodegib in advanced basal-cell carcinoma. N Engl J Med 2012;366(23):2171–9.
33. Dummer R, Guminksi A, Gutzmer R, et al. Long-term efficacy and safety of sonidegib in patients with advanced basal cell carcinoma: 42-month analysis of the phase II randomized, double-blind BOLT study. Br J Dermatol 2020;182(6):1369–78.
34. Sekulic A, Migden MR, Basset-Seguin N, et al. Long-term safety and efficacy of vismodegib in patients with advanced basal cell carcinoma: final update of the pivotal ERIVANCE BCC study. BMC Cancer 2017;17(1):332.
35. De Giorgi V, Scarfi F, Trane L, et al. Treatment of advanced basal cell carcinoma with hedgehog pathway inhibitors: a multidisciplinary expert meeting. Cancers 2021;13(22).
36. Bertrand N, Guerreschi P, Basset-Seguin N, et al. Vismodegib in neoadjuvant treatment of locally advanced basal cell carcinoma: First results of a multicenter, open-label, phase 2 trial (VISMONEO study): Neoadjuvant Vismodegib in Locally Advanced Basal Cell Carcinoma. EClinicalMedicine 2021;35:100844.
37. Stratigos AJ, Garbe C, Dessinioti C, et al. European consensus-based interdisciplinary guideline for invasive cutaneous squamous cell carcinoma: Part 2. Treatment-Update 2023. Eur J Cancer 2023;193:113252.

38. Otsuka A, Dreier J, Cheng PF, et al. Hedgehog pathway inhibitors promote adaptive immune responses in basal cell carcinoma. Clin Cancer Res 2015;21(6): 1289–97.
39. De Giorgi V, Trane L, Savarese I, et al. Lasting response after discontinuation of cemiplimab in a patient with locally advanced basal cell carcinoma. Clin Exp Dermatol 2021;46(8):1612–4.
40. Brodland DG, Zitelli JA. Surgical margins for excision of primary cutaneous squamous cell carcinoma. J Am Acad Dermatol 1992;27(2 Pt 1):241–8.
41. National Comprehensive Cancer Network. Squamous Cell Skin Cancer Version 1.2023. 2023. Available at: https://www.nccn.org/professionals/physician_gls/pdf/squamous.pdf. [Accessed 25 October 2023].
42. Rowe DE, Carroll RJ, Day CL Jr. Prognostic factors for local recurrence, metastasis, and survival rates in squamous cell carcinoma of the skin, ear, and lip. Implications for treatment modality selection. J Am Acad Dermatol 1992;26(6): 976–90.
43. Kofler L, Kofler K, Schulz C, et al. Sentinel lymph node biopsy for high-thickness cutaneous squamous cell carcinoma. Arch Dermatol Res 2021;313(2):119–26.
44. Ilmonen S, Sollamo E, Juteau S, et al. Sentinel lymph node biopsy in high-risk cutaneous squamous cell carcinoma of the head and neck. J Plast Reconstr Aesthetic Surg 2022;75(1):210–6.
45. Allen JE, Stolle LB. Utility of sentinel node biopsy in patients with high-risk cutaneous squamous cell carcinoma. Eur J Surg Oncol 2015;41(2):197–200.
46. Kwon S, Dong ZM, Wu PC. Sentinel lymph node biopsy for high-risk cutaneous squamous cell carcinoma: clinical experience and review of literature. World J Surg Oncol 2011;9:80.
47. Gore SM, Shaw D, Martin RC, et al. Prospective study of sentinel node biopsy for high-risk cutaneous squamous cell carcinoma of the head and neck. Head Neck 2016;38(Suppl 1):E884–9.
48. Schmalbach CE, Ow TJ, Choi KY, et al. American Head and Neck Society position statement on the use of PD-1 inhibitors for treatment of advanced cutaneous squamous cell carcinoma. Head Neck 2023;45(1):32–41.
49. Lansbury L, Bath-Hextall F, Perkins W, et al. Interventions for non-metastatic squamous cell carcinoma of the skin: systematic review and pooled analysis of observational studies. Bmj 2013;347:f6153.
50. Muto P, Pastore F. Radiotherapy in the adjuvant and advanced setting of CSCC. Dermatol Pract Concept 2021;11(Suppl 2):e2021168S.
51. Taylor JM, Dasgeb B, Liem S, et al. High-dose-rate brachytherapy for the treatment of basal and squamous cell carcinomas on sensitive areas of the face: a report of clinical outcomes and acute and subacute toxicities. Adv Radiat Oncol 2021;6(2):100616.
52. Lee CT, Lehrer EJ, Aphale A, et al. Surgical excision, Mohs micrographic surgery, external-beam radiotherapy, or brachytherapy for indolent skin cancer: An international meta-analysis of 58 studies with 21,000 patients. Cancer 2019;125(20): 3582–94.
53. Migden MR, Schmults C, Khushanlani N, et al. 814P Phase II study of cemiplimab in patients with advanced cutaneous squamous cell carcinoma (CSCC): Final analysis from EMPOWER-CSCC-1 groups 1, 2 and 3. Ann Oncol 2022;33:S918–9.
54. Hughes BGM, Munoz-Couselo E, Mortier L, et al. Pembrolizumab for locally advanced and recurrent/metastatic cutaneous squamous cell carcinoma (KEYNOTE-629 study): an open-label, nonrandomized, multicenter, phase II trial. Ann Oncol 2021;32(10):1276–85.

55. Gross ND, Miller DM, Khushalani NI, et al. Neoadjuvant Cemiplimab for Stage II to IV Cutaneous Squamous-Cell Carcinoma. N Engl J Med 2022;387(17):1557–68.
56. Porceddu SV, Bressel M, Poulsen MG, et al. Postoperative concurrent chemoradiotherapy versus postoperative radiotherapy in high-risk cutaneous squamous cell carcinoma of the head and neck: the randomized phase III TROG 05.01 Trial. J Clin Oncol 2018;36(13):1275–83.
57. Andruska N, Fischer-Valuck BW, Mahapatra L, et al. Association between surgical margins larger than 1 cm and overall survival in patients with merkel cell carcinoma. JAMA Dermatol 2021;157(5):540–8.
58. Takagishi SR, Marx TE, Lewis C, et al. Postoperative radiation therapy is associated with a reduced risk of local recurrence among low risk Merkel cell carcinomas of the head and neck. Advances in Radiation Oncology 2016;1(4):244–51.
59. Gupta SG, Wang LC, Peñas PF, et al. Sentinel lymph node biopsy for evaluation and treatment of patients with merkel cell carcinoma: the dana-farber experience and meta-analysis of the literature. Arch Dermatol 2006;142(6):685–90.
60. Kachare SD, Wong JH, Vohra NA, et al. Sentinel lymph node biopsy is associated with improved survival in merkel cell carcinoma. Ann Surg Oncol 2014;21(5):1624–30.
61. Conic RRZ, Ko J, Saridakis S, et al. Sentinel lymph node biopsy in Merkel cell carcinoma: Predictors of sentinel lymph node positivity and association with overall survival. J Am Acad Dermatol 2019;81(2):364–72.
62. Jouary T, Kubica E, Dalle S, et al. Sentinel node status and immunosuppression: recurrence factors in localized Merkel cell carcinoma. Acta Derm Venereol 2015; 95(7):835–40.
63. Servy A, Maubec E, Sugier PE, et al. Merkel cell carcinoma: value of sentinel lymph-node status and adjuvant radiation therapy. Ann Oncol 2016;27(5):914–9.
64. Fields RC, Busam KJ, Chou JF, et al. Recurrence and survival in patients undergoing sentinel lymph node biopsy for merkel cell carcinoma: analysis of 153 patients from a single institution. Ann Surg Oncol 2011;18(9):2529–37.
65. Fojnica A, Ljuca K, Akhtar S, et al. An updated review of the biomarkers of response to immune checkpoint inhibitors in merkel cell carcinoma: merkel cell carcinoma and immunotherapy. Cancers 2023;15(20).
66. Kaufman HL, Russell J, Hamid O, et al. Avelumab in patients with chemotherapy-refractory metastatic Merkel cell carcinoma: a multicentre, single-group, open-label, phase 2 trial. Lancet Oncol 2016;17(10):1374–85.
67. Walker JW, Lebbé C, Grignani G, et al. Efficacy and safety of avelumab treatment in patients with metastatic Merkel cell carcinoma: experience from a global expanded access program. J Immunother Cancer 2020;8(1).
68. Nghiem P, Bhatia S, Lipson EJ, et al. Durable tumor regression and overall survival in patients with advanced merkel cell carcinoma receiving pembrolizumab as first-line therapy. J Clin Oncol 2019;37(9):693–702.
69. Grignani G, Rutkowski P, Lebbe C, et al. 545 A phase 2 study of retifanlimab in patients with advanced or metastatic merkel cell carcinoma (MCC) (POD1UM-201). J ImmunoTherapy Cancer 2021;9(Suppl 2):A574–5.
70. Topalian SL, Bhatia S, Amin A, et al. Neoadjuvant nivolumab for patients with resectable merkel cell carcinoma in the checkMate 358 Trial. J Clin Oncol 2020;38(22):2476–87.
71. Becker JC, Ugurel S, Leiter U, et al. Adjuvant immunotherapy with nivolumab versus observation in completely resected Merkel cell carcinoma (ADMEC-O): disease-free survival results from a randomised, open-label, phase 2 trial. Lancet 2023;402(10404):798–808.

Endoscopic Surgery for Sinonasal and Skull Base Cancer

Alejandra Rodas, MD[a], Leonardo Tariciotti, MD[b],
Biren K. Patel, MBBS[b], Gustavo Pradilla, MD[a,b],
C. Arturo Solares, MD[a,b],*

KEYWORDS

- Endoscopic endonasal surgery • Sinonasal cancer • Skull base cancer
- Skull base reconstruction

KEY POINTS

- Endoscopic endonasal surgery has become the first-line treatment for multiple early-stage sinonasal and skull base malignancies.
- Studies have shown endoscopic endonasal procedures are linked to fewer postoperative complications and shorter length of hospital stay.
- Although endoscopic endonasal surgery does not follow the oncologic principle of en-bloc resection, piecemeal resection has not been shown to influence recurrence or survival outcomes.

INTRODUCTION

Improvements in endoscopic technologies coupled with close collaboration of otolaryngologists and neurosurgeons have been key in the development of endoscopic endonasal surgery. Once limited to benign pathologies, endoscopic techniques are now considered the first line of treatment in selected cases of malignant sinonasal and skull base tumors.[1] Large cohort studies have reported that adenocarcinoma, olfactory neuroblastoma (ONB), and squamous cell carcinoma (SCC) are among the most common pathologies treated endoscopically.[2–4] Moreover, these studies noted endoscopic resection was primarily used in cases of T1 and T2 tumors, while the majority of T3 and T4 tumors relied on endoscopic-assisted craniofacial resection.[2–4]

[a] Department of Otolaryngology – Head and Neck Surgery, Emory University Hospital Midtown, 9th Floor, Medical Office Tower, 550 Peachtree NE, Atlanta, GA 30308, USA;
[b] Department of Neurosurgery, Emory Faculty Office Building, 49 Jesse Hill Jr. Drive SE, Atlanta, GA 30303, USA
* Corresponding author. Emory University Hospital Midtown, 9th Floor, Medical Office Tower, 550 Peachtree Street Northeast, Atlanta, GA 30308.
E-mail address: csolare@emory.edu

Surg Oncol Clin N Am 33 (2024) 735–746
https://doi.org/10.1016/j.soc.2024.04.007
surgonc.theclinics.com

A major concern related to endoscopic endonasal approaches (EEAs) was the inability to attain en-bloc tumor excision with negative margins. However, it has been proven that piecemeal resection does not jeopardize survival outcomes.[5] Complications related to traditional open approaches, such as meningitis and wound dehiscence, are reduced in rate. The endonasal corridor provides a more direct access to the tumor, minimizing manipulation of critical neurovascular structures. This has correlated with reduced postoperative pain and length of hospital stay.[2]

As surgical teams gained more experience and instrumentation improved, the boundaries of EEAs became broader. A series of expanded approaches have been developed to deal with different skull base regions.[6,7] Previously described only for the management of midline lesions, endoscopic surgery now offers approaches that target the paramedian skull base, minimizing retraction of vascular and neural structures within the coronal plane.[8]

PREOPERATIVE AND INTRAOPERATIVE CONSIDERATIONS

Preoperative imaging[9] and a protocol of imaging interpretation should be followed, establishing the lesion's location, encasement of the internal carotid artery (ICA), cavernous sinus involvement, displacement of cranial nerves (CNs), perineural spread, and intra-orbital invasion.[10] Contraindications for endoscopic approach include tumors causing bone erosion at the lateral, anterior, or inferior walls of the maxillary sinus, as well as those significantly infiltrating the frontal sinus, nasal floor, or intracranial compartment.[6] Virtual reality models have been developed to allow preoperative surgical planning, recreating the surgical corridor and target lesion. Imaging studies can render a 3-dimensional (3D) reconstruction of the patient's anatomy in cases of endoscopic surgery targeting the craniovertebral junction. This allowed establishing the proximity of the ICA and the extent of resection required to safely expose the odontoid.[11]

In endoscopic surgery, bleeding can significantly influence the surgeon's performance; hence, intraoperative preparation should include pro-hemostatic medical interventions such as controlled hypotension, nasal vasoconstrictors, head elevation, and tranexamic acid.[12] Additional equipment that reduces the interruption caused by constant bleeding includes endoscope washing sheaths and the microdebrider, which offers continuous suction while cutting and removing tissue. Setting up intranasal coagulation devices such as the endoscopic bipolar cautery or suction coagulator is particularly important in the context of tumor resection since lesions can be highly vascular.

Success rate in tumor resection has been reported to be higher when adequately angled endoscopes and instruments are used.[12] Endoscopic surgery for cancer treatment often involves 2 surgeons: one handling the endoscope and the other manipulating instruments and suction. Articulated stands have been developed to hold the scope, augmenting the ease of single-surgeon operation. Nonetheless, there are limits to what a single surgeon can accomplish, and an experienced surgical team is highly advised. Camera definition has significantly progressed in the past decade, now offering 4K image quality and 3D endoscopy.[12] These advancements have improved the identification of structures and depth perception. Intraoperatively, imaging-based navigation systems are also strongly advised, as they guide the surgeon through distorted anatomy while avoiding injury of critical vascular structures, ensuring adequate resection, and potentially reducing operative time. Moreover, neurovascular morbidity is reduced by the use of carotid Doppler and neuromonitoring CNs.

Anatomy

The anterior skull base corresponds to the roof of the nasal cavities and is formed by the ethmoid, frontal, and sphenoid bones. It is bounded anteriorly by the posterior table of frontal sinus, laterally on both sides by the junction of lamina papyracea and fovea ethmoidalis, and posteriorly by the tuberculum sellae.[13] The cribriform plate and crista galli are encountered in the midline and have superolateral continuity with the fovea ethmoidalis. The cribriform plate is perforated, allowing the olfactory bulbs to synapse with olfactory fila that spread across the nasal septum and superior and middle turbinates. In the ethmoidal roof, 2 major arteries can be identified.[14] The anterior ethmoidal artery crosses posterior to the nasofrontal recess while the posterior ethmoidal artery forms its trajectory at the border of the planum sphenoidale.

The sphenoid sinus comprehends a group of critical landmarks, including the sella turcica, middle clivus and clival recess, the paraclival ICA, and the optic nerve prominence. The parasellar region is consistent with the cavernous sinus.[14] Drilling the lateral wall of the sphenoid, CN VI can be observed running behind the paraclival carotid and toward the cavernous sinus. CN III, IV, and the ophthalmic branch of the trigeminal nerve can be seen coursing toward the superior orbital fissure.

In the coronal plane, endoscopic access to the middle cranial fossa and lateral aspect of the cavernous sinus is possible through alternate routes. Understanding the anatomic relationship between the maxillary sinus, pterygopalatine fossa (PPF), and infratemporal fossa (ITF) is crucial. The orbital floor serves as the maxillary sinus's roof and houses the maxillary branch of the trigeminal nerve. Posteriorly, the sinus is limited by the PPF, which contains the internal maxillary artery and pterygopalatine ganglion. Under the middle cranial fossa, the ITF lies lateral to the PPF, separated by the pterygomaxillary fissure, and contains the parapharyngeal and masticator spaces.[8] The vidian nerve, running through the pterygoid canal on the floor of the sphenoid sinus, serves as a critical landmark for horizontal petrosal ICA.

The posterior skull base is accessed via the dorsum sellae, frontal aspect of the clivus, and craniovertebral junction. The clivus forms the anterior margin of the foramen magnum and is divided into the sellar, sphenoidal, and nasopharyngeal segments. The petroclival fissure and foramen lacerum lie on its lateral aspect, separating it from the temporal bone and petrous apex.[13,15]

ENDOSCOPIC APPROACHES

At the initial stages of an endoscopic procedure, the field might be completely obstructed by the lesion. Gradual debulking of the tumor will clear the path and anatomic landmarks can be identified. Maxillary and sphenoidal sinusotomies serve both for control of the tumor and orientation. The lesion must be traced back to its origin, and surgical margins can be analyzed as frozen sections to establish the limits of resection.[2] The range of the exposure is determined by the tumor's location. Frequently, a binostril approach will be required, and this is accomplished by resecting the posterior two-thirds of the nasal septum. Additionally, specific approaches are required for pathologies with characteristic growth patterns.

Transsphenoidal Approach

The transsphenoidal approach is the workhorse in pituitary tumor resection. Substituting transnasal microscopic approaches, endoscopic endonasal surgery proved to be more effective in reducing rates of cerebrospinal fluid (CSF) leaks, meningitis, operative time, length of hospital stay, and postsurgical endocrinopathies.[16–18] Phan and colleagues[17] reported endoscopic transsphenoidal surgery was associated with a higher remission rate in noninvasive macroadenomas, when compared to those treated microsurgically.

This approach deals with the complexity of the sphenoid sinus, and careful attention is required preoperatively when assessing its size, shape, and variable pneumatization.[19] A wide sphenoidotomy is performed and the intersinus septum is removed to allow binostril access to the sellar region.[6] The sphenoid rostrum is also resected to expose the inferior margin of the dissection, although careful attention is needed during this step as the vascularity of the nasoseptal flap (NSF) should not be compromised. Ideally, the edges of the sphenoidotomy must be resected in a centripetal manner in order to achieve a good angle of maneuverability within the sinus. The approach must ensure sufficient endoscopic control and clear visualization of the parasellar carotids, sella, optic nerves, and optic-carotid recesses.

Transcribriform Approach

A transcribriform approach is required for access to midline lesions such as olfactory groove meningiomas, ethmoid adenocarcinomas, and ONBs.[7,20] Depending on the extension of the tumor, the approach can be performed unilaterally or bilaterally. A wider endoscopic armamentarium is required to successfully accomplish gross total resection since frontal sinus manipulation, a crucial step of the approach, relies on angled instrumentation and endoscopes. Generally associated with postoperative olfaction dysfunction, patients undergoing this procedure should be informed about the risk.[9]

Following a total ethmoidectomy, sphenoidotomy, and posterior and superior septectomy, the transcribriform approach consists of a modified Lothrop procedure, cauterization of the ethmoidal arteries, and frontal and bilateral osteotomies.[7] After the frontal sinusotomy is performed, the posterior table of the frontal sinus can be easily discerned, and it marks the site for the frontal osteotomy.[20] Lateral osteotomies are performed through high-speed drilling with the lamina papyracea as the lateral limit. These osteotomies border anteriorly with the frontal osteotomy and posteriorly with the planum sphenoidale (**Fig. 1**). If the tumor extends more posterior, it is feasible to widen the bony keyhole margins toward the tuberculum sellae.[20] The crista galli is then resected and the dura is incised if an intracranial component is present.

Transpterygoid Approach

The endoscopic transpterygoid approach is a less invasive alternative for lesions involving the lateral cavernous sinus, Meckel's cave, petrous apex, and petroclival synchondrosis.[21] This approach is initiated with a maxillary antrostomy, bilateral sphenoidotomies, and removal of the sphenoid sinus floor.[8] The sphenopalatine artery is then identified and coagulated, and the posterior wall of the maxillary sinus is removed, exposing the sphenopalatine ganglion (**Fig. 2**).[21] Sacrificing the pharyngeal artery and nerve, the ganglion can be mobilized laterally, and the pterygoid canal (vidian canal) is identified. Removal of the medial pterygoid process between the pterygoid canal and foramen rotundum is required.[13] The vidian nerve's trajectory is then followed posteriorly until the transition between laceral and paraclival ICA is met. The petrous apex can be accessed by skeletonizing and mobilizing the ICA. Else, only tumors that expand the petrous apex can be resected through a transsphenoidal approach. Such would be the case of cholesterol granulomas.[7] In addition, the eustachian tube may be removed to expose the petroclival synchondrosis completely. Meckel's cave, which houses pathologies such as invasive adenoid cystic carcinomas, meningiomas, and schwannomas, is accessed through the quadrangular space, which is limited inferiorly and medially by the petrous and paraclival ICA, respectively.[8]

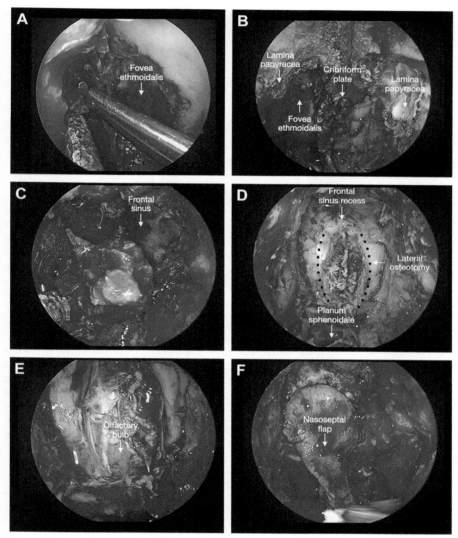

Fig. 1. Transcribriform approach consists of (*A*) bilateral ethmoidectomy, (*B*) complete exposure of the anterior skull base, (*C*) modified Lothrop procedure, (*D*) cribriform plate resection, (*E*) durotomy and exposure of the olfactory bulb, and (*F*) reconstruction of the skull base defect.

Transclival Approach

The transclival approach starts with removal of the vomer and inferior wall of the sphenoid sinus. The vidian nerves, located at the level of the sphenoid sinus floor, are critical landmarks that help track the location of the clival carotid arteries and represent the lateral limit of the approach at this level. Moving posteriorly, the transclival exposure is typically limited laterally by the interdural CN VI (**Fig. 3**),[7] but the limits of exposure can be widened by neuromonitoring the location of the nerve. The upper clivus is formed by the posterior clinoid processes and dorsum sellae. High-speed drilling of

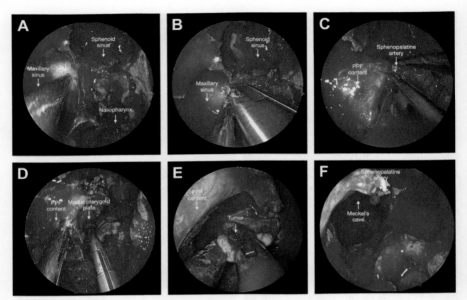

Fig. 2. Transpterygoid approach for resection of a right Meckel's cave schwannoma. (*A*) A wide maxillary antrostomy and bilateral sphenoidotomy are performed. (*B*) The posterior wall of the maxillary sinus is resected. (*C*) The sphenopalatine artery is coagulated. (*D*) The pterygoid plates are drilled out. (*E*) Dissection and lateralization of the pterygopalatine fossa's contents expose the lesion on Meckel's cave, and (*F*) gross total resection is achieved. PPF, pterygopalatine fossa.

the sphenoidal clivus between the paraclival ICA projections allows access to the prepontine cistern, exposing the basilar artery, anterior inferior cerebellar artery, and CNs III and VI.[13,14] The inferior clivus is exposed by reflecting the pharyngobasilar fascia, followed by detachment of the longus colli and longus capitis muscles. Drilling of this clival segment will gain access to the foramen magnum, hypoglossal canal, occipital condyles, anterior arch of C1, and craniocervical junction.[14] Removing the anterior arch of C1 allows exposure of the dens.[13] The inferior limit of transclival exposure at this level is determined by the hard palate.[7]

SINONASAL AND SKULL BASE ONCOLOGIC PATHOLOGIES
Squamous Cell Carcinoma

SCCs constitute the most common malignancy of the nose and paranasal sinuses.[22] The American Joint Committee on Cancer divides sinonasal carcinomas based on the site where they originated (nasal cavity, ethmoid sinuses, or maxillary sinuses).[23] Patients with nasal cavity SCC often develop symptoms earlier whereas tumors of the paranasal sinuses are typically asymptomatic on their initial stages, causing later diagnosis and the need for aggressive management. SCCs are locally aggressive, fast-growing tumors with a high rate of local and regional recurrence. They most frequently arise from the maxillary sinus, and more than 80% of patients whose SCC arises from this location present with stage T3 to T4 disease.[24] Depending on its location, SCCs can extend to nearby structures including the oral cavity, PPF, ITF, anterior skull base, intracranial compartment, and orbit. The anterior cranial fossa can also be involved following perineural spread on CNs.[23]

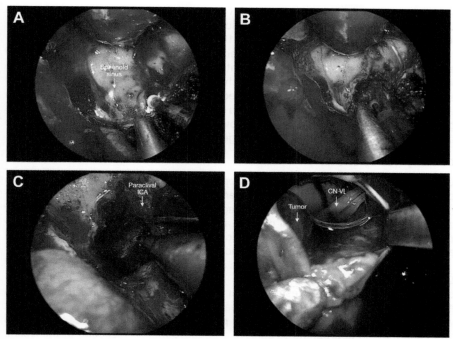

Fig. 3. Petroclival lesion resection. (*A*) Bilateral sphenoidotomy is followed by (*B*) clival drilling. (*C*) The paraclival ICA is skeletonized and gently mobilized laterally. (*D*) Dura is incised, and the tumor is observed in close contact with CN VI. CN, cranial nerve; ICA, internal carotid artery.

The treatment of sinonasal SCCs consists of surgical resection and adjuvant intensity-modulated radiotherapy (IMRT).[23] Surgical treatment should aim for negative margin resection, with the least damage to surrounding structures. Depending on the extent of the lesion, complementary open field procedures such as orbital exenteration, maxillectomy, and neck dissection may be needed. Survival rates have shown similar outcomes between endoscopic and craniofacial resection,[25] yet these studies depend on a high selection bias that consider the limitations of the endoscopic route. Stage T4 SCC of the nasal cavity and tumor size larger than 2 cm are both associated with increased rates of cervical lymph node compromise.[26] Thus, radiation to the neck is encouraged in patients with late-stage tumors (T3–T4) as this reduces the risk of regional recurrence.[23]

Adenocarcinoma

Sinonasal adenocarcinomas can be classified as salivary-type, intestinal-type, or non-intestinal–type.[27] Sinonasal adenocarcinoma most commonly arise from the ethmoid sinus (85%) and olfactory cleft (13%).[6] Due to physical proximity, these tumors involve the anterior skull base with greater frequency than SCCs.[22] Poor prognostic factors include advanced tumor stage, tumor volume, positive nodal status, positive surgical margins, poor histologic differentiation, and invasion of the brain, orbit, ITF, or sphenoid.[10]

These tumors are standardly treated through surgical resection, which, based on the extension of the lesion, can be achieved through EEAs or an open approach such as midfacial degloving or lateral rhinotomy.[10] Since occupational exposure to wood and leather dust is related to the development of adenocarcinoma, lesions can be multifocal and bilateral ethmoid resection is recommended.[6] Meccariello and colleagues[5] performed a pooled analysis of 1826 patients which demonstrated consistently higher disease-free survival, local recurrence-free survival, and overall survival across all stages in patients who underwent endoscopic resection, compared to those who were treated with an open approach. Additionally, they found that advanced stage and open approach were associated with higher rates of major complication as well as local relapses. Hospital stay was significantly shorter within the endoscopic group.[5] Postoperative IMRT has been shown to improve survival rates in high-grade adenocarcinomas independent of the stage.[6]

Olfactory Neuroblastoma

ONBs are rare malignancies that arise from the olfactory neuroepithelium, which is distributed along the cribriform plate, superior aspect of the nasal septum, and superior and middle turbinates. The Kadish staging system divides ONBs based on their extension through the paranasal cavities and skull base. Diaz and colleagues[28] reported this staging system had prognostic significance in relation to 5-year survival and combined regional and local recurrence.

The standard of treatment of ONB relies on surgical resection and adjuvant IMRT.[9] Devaiah and colleagues[29] noted surgery had significantly more disease-free outcomes and better survival rates than other modalities of treatment. ONB appears as a polypoid mass positioned high in the nasal cavity. As most ONB are in close contact with the anterior skull base at the time of presentation, performing a transcribriform approach may be appropriate to achieve a negative margin resection of the lesion, including invaded dura, olfactory bulb, and any small intracranial component. Castelnuovo and colleagues[6] stated surgical excision of ONB should include the dura along with the ipsilateral olfactory bulb with the purpose of achieving free margins and properly staging each case. Bilateral olfactory bulbs are resected only if there is evidence of tumor extension to the contralateral side.[6] Orbital wall invasion should be assessed and treated accordingly through periorbital dissection. Moreover, an open approach may be of use if the intracranial portion of the tumor surpasses the limits of what can be debulked through the endonasal route.

Over the past 2 decades, a shifting trend has been observed, favoring endoscopic surgery over open transcranial approaches. Devaiah and colleagues[29] reported endoscopic surgery had better survival rates than the open surgery group. This shift could also be related to the outstanding advancements in the endoscopic instrument catalog and the decreased rate of postoperative complications. Nonetheless, surgical planning should proceed with caution. ONBs tend to present with late recurrence and results endorsing endoscopic surgery could be influenced by the discrepancy in median follow-up time and Kadish stage.[6,29] Hence, long-term surveillance is required after treatment.[6]

Chordoma

Chordomas are malignant and locally destructive tumors that arise from notochord remnants. They are slow-growing lesions that constitute merely 1% of intracranial tumors. They mainly arise in the axial skeleton, affecting the skull base at the level of the clivus.[30] They have also been reported to arise from the petrous apex, although this presentation is rare.[15] Chordomas are well-defined lesions that erode bony structures. Clival chordomas, through their expansive growth pattern, tend to generate CN III and VI palsies, hydrocephalus, and sensorimotor deficits.[30] On computed tomography scan, chordomas appear as a well-circumscribed mass with lytic destruction of the clivus. They are hyperintense on T2-weighted MRI and hypointense on T1-weighted MRI.[15] Surgery is the primary treatment for these lesions and the extent of resection dictates the effectiveness of postsurgical radiotherapy.[1]

As a midline skull base tumor, the endoscopic endonasal route is ideal for resection of chordomas. Gross total resection has been reported to range from 50% to 90%, depending on the experience of the surgeon and the extension of the lesion.[1,30] For chordomas affecting the petroclival region, a pure EEA may not be the best choice as this would require mobilization of the petrous carotid. The risk of vascular injury can be minimized by shaping a contralateral transmaxillary corridor.[1]

RECONSTRUCTION TECHNIQUES

Gross total resection of sinonasal malignancies through EEAs can lead to large skull base dura defects or dehiscence of critical neurovascular structures. Reconstruction aims at recreating the physical separation between the cranial vault and sinonasal cavity, while also enduring the postoperative insult that radiotherapy inflicts. A vascularized flap must be pursued in such cases as they heal in shorter time and allow prompt adjuvant therapy initiation. A multilayer reconstruction technique is preferred.[6] In our experience, the first layer corresponds to dural repair with synthetic dura substitutes positioned through an inlay or onlay technique. Autologous materials such as fascia lata can also be used for this purpose. The second step consists of placing the vascularized flap over the defect, ensuring water-tight closure. Positioning of the flap must be done with vigilance, preventing torsion or transection of the flap's vascular pedicle as well as inadvertent displacement of the first layer. Finally, cellulose strips are placed along the edges of the flap and the nasal cavity is firmly packed.

Local Flaps

Several vascularized endonasal flaps can be adequately used for skull base reconstruction, reducing morbidity related to external incisions. The NSF is the most common reconstruction technique in endoscopic endonasal skull base surgery. Supplied by the posterior nasal artery, a branch of the sphenopalatine artery, this flap offers a large coverage area with great arc of rotation.[31] The NSF is ideal for reconstruction of anterior and middle skull base defects as well as clival and parasellar skull base.[32] It is harvested from the axial plane, dissecting the mucoperichondrium and mucoperiosteum away from the nasal septum. The inferior incision can be extended into the nasal cavity floor, depending on the magnitude of the defect. The nasoseptal rescue flap is a modified version in which the pedicle is dissected but not the rest of the paddle. It helps preserve the vascularity of the flap in cases where the NSF is not routinely harvested due to low probability of CSF leak, as is the case of pituitary surgery.[32]

The inferior turbinate flap is a local pedicled flap that might be used alone or as complement of the NSF. Its vascularization comes from the inferior turbinate artery, a branch of the posterior lateral nasal artery. The inferior turbinate artery is harvested on its entirety, leaving it pedicled on its posterolateral aspect. Its arc of rotation is reduced, compared to that of the NSF, making clival or sellar defects its main targets.[31] The posterior pedicle lateral nasal wall flap, on the other hand, is composed from the inferolateral wall and the floor of the nasal cavity. This significantly bigger flap paddle makes it ideal for rotation into the planum sphenoidale, nasopharynx, and orbital apex.[32] The middle turbinate flap can be used for reconstruction of the sella, planum sphenoidale, and fovea ethmoidalis. Its arc of rotation is enhanced by dissecting the flap's pedicle toward the sphenopalatine foramen.[31,32]

Regional Flaps

Regional flaps are useful when intranasal options have been exhausted or involved by the tumor itself. The temporoparietal fascia flap is a vascularized regional flap comprised by the fascial layer underlying the subcutaneous tissue at the temporoparietal region. The paddle, pedicled on the superficial temporal artery, is tunneled through a transpterygoid corridor.[32] This flap is optimal for reconstruction at the anterior and middle skull base, including clival and parasellar defects.[33] Fortes and colleagues[33] reported adequate vascularization and integration of the temporoparietal fascia flap in 2 patients treated for recurrent clival chordoma.

The pericranial flap is a fascial regional flap, with vascular flow provided by the supraorbital and supratrochlear arteries.[32] It can be harvested through a coronal incision or endoscopically. The flap can be raised unilaterally, restricting dissection at the midline. This way, the contralateral side is saved as backup for future procedures.[34] The harvested fascia is used for anterior skull base reconstruction, tunneling the flap through a small osteotomy at the nasion. A Draf III frontal sinusotomy must be performed to allow space for the flap.

Free Tissue Transfer

Patients who have undergone wide tumor resections or are affected by treatment complications such as osteomyelitis and osteoradionecrosis must be treated with vascularized reconstructive flaps. Free flaps are ideal for this purpose, providing a large bulk of tissue anastomosed to a strong blood supply. Harvested from a site distinct to the primary pathology, these flaps are not devitalized by prior treatment. Available donor sites include the transverse rectus abdominis muscle, radial forearm, and the anterolateral thigh.[35,36] The paddle of tissue must be harvested with a sufficiently long vascular pedicle, which will later be anastomosed with the facial vessels at the neck. A safe corridor must be fashioned for transposition of the flap into the sinonasal cavity. This can be achieved through a Caldwell-Luc/buccal space corridor, prevertebral corridor, transpterygoid/parapharyngeal corridor, among others.[37]

SUMMARY

Endoscopic endonasal surgery has been continuously evolving, and the list of indications has broadened accordingly. Improvements in camera quality and instrument selection, coupled with the growing expertise of each surgical team, have made feasible the endoscopic management of complex sinonasal and skull base malignant tumors. Moreover, oncologic reports have shown promising results, pointing at better disease-specific survival rates among patients treated endoscopically.

CLINICS CARE POINTS

- Surgical planning requires a detailed evaluation of preoperative images, establishing the extent of the lesion and neurovascular involvement.

- Approach selection is based on the tumor's size, invasion pattern, and disposition in relation to critical neurovascular structures.

- Working with a multidisciplinary team is crucial for the management and follow-up of patients with sinonasal and skull base malignancies.

DISCLOSURE

No external funding was received. C.A. Solares serves as a consultant for Medtronic. G. Pradilla serves as a consultant for Stryker Corporation. A. Rodas, L. Tariciotti, and B.K. Patel have no conflict of interest to declare.

REFERENCES

1. Snyderman CH, Carrau RL, Kassam AB, et al. Endoscopic skull base surgery: principles of endonasal oncological surgery. J Surg Oncol 2008;97(8):658–64.
2. Castelnuovo P, Battaglia P, Turri-Zanoni M, et al. Endoscopic endonasal surgery for malignancies of the anterior cranial base. World Neurosurg 2014;82(6 Suppl): S22–31.
3. Nicolai P, Battaglia P, Bignami M, et al. Endoscopic surgery for malignant tumors of the sinonasal tract and adjacent skull base: a 10-year experience. Am J Rhinol 2008;22(3):308–16.
4. Hanna E, DeMonte F, Ibrahim S, et al. Endoscopic resection of sinonasal cancers with and without craniotomy: oncologic results. Arch Otolaryngol Head Neck Surg 2009;135(12):1219–24.
5. Meccariello G, Deganello A, Choussy O, et al. Endoscopic nasal versus open approach for the management of sinonasal adenocarcinoma: A pooled-analysis of 1826 patients. Head Neck 2016;38(Suppl 1):E2267–74.
6. Castelnuovo P, Turri-Zanoni M, Battaglia P, et al. Sinonasal malignancies of anterior skull base: histology-driven treatment strategies. Otolaryngol Clin North Am 2016;49(1):183–200.
7. Zwagerman NT, Zenonos G, Lieber S, et al. Endoscopic transnasal skull base surgery: pushing the boundaries. J Neuro Oncol 2016;130(2):319–30.
8. de Lara D, Ditzel Filho LF, Prevedello DM, et al. Endonasal endoscopic approaches to the paramedian skull base. World Neurosurg 2014;82(6 Suppl): S121–9.
9. Ivan ME, Han SJ, Aghi MK. Tumors of the anterior skull base. Expert Rev Neurother 2014;14(4):425–38.
10. Lund VJ, Chisholm EJ, Takes RP, et al. Evidence for treatment strategies in sinonasal adenocarcinoma. Head Neck 2012;34(8):1168–78.
11. Filimonov A, Zeiger J, Goldrich D, et al. Virtual reality surgical planning for endoscopic endonasal approaches to the craniovertebral junction. Am J Otolaryngol Jan-Feb 2022;43(1):103219.
12. Khanwalkar AR, Welch KC. Updates in techniques for improved visualization in sinus surgery. Curr Opin Otolaryngol Head Neck Surg 2021;29(1):9–20.
13. Solari D, Chiaramonte C, Di Somma A, et al. Endoscopic anatomy of the skull base explored through the nose. World Neurosurg 2014;82(6 Suppl):S164–70.
14. Patel CR, Fernandez-Miranda JC, Wang WH, et al. Skull Base Anatomy. Otolaryngol Clin North Am 2016;49(1):9–20.
15. Hofmann E, Prescher A. The clivus: anatomy, normal variants and imaging pathology. Clin Neuroradiol 2012;22(2):123–39.
16. Rotenberg B, Tam S, Ryu WH, et al. Microscopic versus endoscopic pituitary surgery: a systematic review. Laryngoscope 2010;120(7):1292–7.
17. Phan K, Xu J, Reddy R, et al. Endoscopic endonasal versus microsurgical transsphenoidal approach for growth hormone-secreting pituitary adenomas-systematic review and meta-analysis. World Neurosurg 2017;97:398–406.

18. Martinez-Perez R, Silveira-Bertazzo G, Albonette-Felicio T, et al. Chapter 23 - Extended transsphenoidal surgery. In: Honegger J, Reincke M, Petersenn S, editors. Pituitary tumors. Cambridge, MA: Academic Press; 2021. p. 327–41.
19. El Hadi U, El Hadi N, Hosri J, et al. Tips and tricks to safely perform an endoscopic endonasal trans-sphenoidal pituitary surgery: a surgeon's checklist. Indian J Otolaryngol Head Neck Surg 2023;75(4):4116–24.
20. Liu JK, Christiano LD, Patel SK, et al. Surgical nuances for removal of olfactory groove meningiomas using the endoscopic endonasal transcribriform approach. Neurosurg Focus 2011;30(5):E3.
21. Singh AK, Patel BK, Darshan HR, et al. Endoscopic transpterygoid corridor for petroclival tumors: case series and technical nuances. Neurol India 2023;71(6):1159–66.
22. Mani N, Shah JP. Squamous cell carcinoma and its variants. Adv Oto-Rhino-Laryngol 2020;84:124–36.
23. Leonard CG, Padhye V, Witterick IJ. Management of squamous cell carcinomas of the skull-base. J Neuro Oncol 2020;150(3):377–86.
24. Dubal PM, Bhojwani A, Patel TD, et al. Squamous cell carcinoma of the maxillary sinus: A population-based analysis. Laryngoscope 2016;126(2):399–404.
25. Harvey RJ, Winder M, Parmar P, et al. Endoscopic skull base surgery for sinonasal malignancy. Otolaryngol Clin North Am 2011;44(5):1081–140.
26. Janik S, Gramberger M, Kadletz L, et al. Impact of anatomic origin of primary squamous cell carcinomas of the nasal cavity and ethmoidal sinus on clinical outcome. Eur Arch Oto-Rhino-Laryngol 2018;275(9):2363–71.
27. Leivo I. Sinonasal Adenocarcinoma: Update on classification, immunophenotype and molecular features. Head Neck Pathol 2016;10(1):68–74.
28. Diaz EM Jr, Johnigan RH, Pero C, et al. Olfactory neuroblastoma: the 22-year experience at one comprehensive cancer center. Head Neck 2005;27(2):138–49.
29. Devaiah AK, Andreoli MT. Treatment of esthesioneuroblastoma: a 16-year meta-analysis of 361 patients. Laryngoscope 2009;119(7):1412–6.
30. Mendenhall WM, Mendenhall CM, Lewis SB, et al. Skull base chordoma. Head Neck 2005;27(2):159–65.
31. Bhatki AM, Pant H, Snyderman CH, et al. Reconstruction of the cranial base after endonasal skull base surgery: Local tissue flaps. Operat Tech Otolaryngol Head Neck Surg 2010;21(1):74–82.
32. Tang IP, Carrau RL, Otto BA, et al. Technical nuances of commonly used vascularised flaps for skull base reconstruction. J Laryngol Otol 2015;129(8):752–61.
33. Fortes FS, Carrau RL, Snyderman CH, et al. Transpterygoid transposition of a temporoparietal fascia flap: a new method for skull base reconstruction after endoscopic expanded endonasal approaches. Laryngoscope 2007;117(6):970–6.
34. Kim GG, Hang AX, Mitchell CA, et al. Pedicled extranasal flaps in skull base reconstruction. Adv Oto-Rhino-Laryngol 2013;74:71–80.
35. Bell EB, Cohen ER, Sargi Z, et al. Free tissue reconstruction of the anterior skull base: A review. World J Otorhinolaryngol Head Neck Surg 2020;6(2):132–6.
36. Wang W, Vincent A, Sokoya M, et al. Free-flap reconstruction of skull base and orbital defects. Semin Plast Surg 2019;33(1):72–7.
37. Dang RP, Roland LT, Sharon JD, et al. Pedicle corridors and vessel options for free flap reconstruction following endoscopic endonasal skull base surgery: a systematic review. J Neurol Surg B Skull Base 2021;82(2):196–201.

Update on the Treatment of Salivary Gland Carcinomas

Danielle M. Gillard, MD[a], Zainab Farzal, MD, MPH[a,b],
William R. Ryan, MD[a,*]

KEYWORDS

- Salivary gland carcinoma • Salivary gland malignancy • Mucoepidermoid carcinoma
- Adenoid cystic carcinoma • Acinic cell carcinoma

KEY POINTS

- Salivary gland carcinomas (SGC), although low incidence, are comprised of a variety of histologic subtypes, which can make preoperative diagnosis challenging.
- Currently, MRI is the modality of choice for preoperative evaluation of salivary gland malignancies.
- Upfront surgery with removal of the primary tumor has been shown to have better survival than upfront radiotherapy; however, the management of the clinically negative neck with upfront surgery versus radiation is an area of debate.
- Reconstruction of parotidectomy SGC defects has been shown to improve cosmetic outcomes and decreases the risk of postoperative Frey syndrome.
- Currently, chemotherapy and immunotherapy have a limited role in the management of SGC.

BACKGROUND AND EPIDEMIOLOGY

Salivary gland carcinomas (SGC) are rare, comprising 5% of all head and neck cancers,[1] with an incidence of approximately 1 per 100,000 per year.[2] Despite their relative rarity, SGCs comprise a large variety of distinct subtypes with unique courses, prognoses, and management paradigms. The World Health Organization currently recognizes more than 20 different subtypes of SGC and 15 subtypes of benign tumors (**Table 1**).[3–5] The most common subtypes in the major and minor salivary glands are mucoepidermoid carcinoma, with an incidence of 0.285 per 100,000, and adenoid cystic carcinoma (ACC), with an incidence of 0.130 per 100,000.[1,6–8] Squamous cell carcinoma is also common, with an incidence of 0.183 per 100,000, although these are usually cutaneous squamous cell carcinoma metastases. Such metastases are

[a] Department of Otolaryngology–Head and Neck Surgery, University of California San Francisco, San Francisco, CA, USA; [b] Department of Otolaryngology Head and Neck Surgery, University of Texas Southwestern Medical Center, 5323 Harry Hines Boulevard, Dallas, TX 75390-9035, USA
* Corresponding author. Otolaryngology–Head and Neck Surgery, University of California San Francisco, 2233 Post Street, 3rd Floor, San Francisco, CA 94115.
E-mail address: William.ryan@ucsf.edu

Surg Oncol Clin N Am 33 (2024) 747–760
https://doi.org/10.1016/j.soc.2024.04.008
1055-3207/24/© 2024 Elsevier Inc. All rights reserved.
surgonc.theclinics.com

Table 1
Subtypes of salivary gland carcinoma

World Health Organization Classification of Benign and Malignant Tumors of the Salivary Glands	
Mucoepidermoid carcinoma	Pleomorphic adenoma
Adenoid cystic carcinoma	Basal cell adenoma
Acinic cell carcinoma	Warthin tumor
Secretory carcinoma	Oncocytoma
Microsecretory adenocarcinoma	Salivary gland myoepithelioma
Polymorphous adenocarcinoma	Canalicular adenoma
Hyalinizing clear cell carcinoma	Cystadenoma of salivary gland
Basal cell adenocarcinoma	Ductal papillomas
Intraductal carcinoma	Sialadenoma papilliferum
Salivary duct carcinoma	Lymphadenoma
Myoepithelial carcinoma	Sebaceous adenoma
Epithelial-myoepithelial carcinoma	Intercalated duct adenoma and hyperplasia
Mucinous adenocarcinoma	Striated duct adenoma
Sclerosing microcystic adenocarcinoma	Sclerosing polycystic adenoma
Carcinoma ex pleomorphic adenoma	Keratocystoma
Carcinosarcoma of the salivary glands	
Sebaceous adenocarcinoma	
Lymphoepithelial carcinoma	
Squamous cell carcinoma	
Sialoblastoma	
Salivary carcinoma, not otherwise specified and emerging entities	

Adapted from World Health Organization Classification of Head and Neck Tumors.[4,5]

confused with squamous variants of mucoepidermoid carcinoma.[1,6] The incidence also varies per subsite. Parotid neoplasms have the lowest malignancy rate of about 25%, followed by 43% for submandibular glands and 82% for minor salivary glands.[9] There are no clear risk factors for the development of SGC, although ionizing radiation has been implicated.[9,10] The common risk factors for head and neck carcinoma, alcohol and smoking, have not demonstrated a clear relationship with SGC. A correlation does exist between smoking and the benign neoplasm papillary lymphomatous cystadenoma, also known as Warthin tumor.[11]

Pleomorphic adenoma is the most common benign salivary gland histology that has a small, but real risk for malignant transformation to carcinoma ex pleomorphic adenoma.[12,13] Traditionally, it was shown that the risk of malignant transformation was approximately 1.5% for the first 5 years of diagnosis, but increases to 10% 15 years after diagnosis.[12] Given this possible risk, traditional recommendations have been to perform surgical resection of the benign lesion to avoid malignant transformation. However, newer studies show the risk of malignant transformation for pleomorphic adenoma, and especially recurrent pleomorphic adenoma, is likely much lower than originally believed. In a Danish national health care database study of 5497 patients over a 25-year period, the malignant transformation for primary pleomorphic adenoma was 0.25% and for recurrent pleomorphic adenoma was 3.3%.[14] Similarly, in a Dutch national health care database study of 3506 patients, malignant transformation occurred in 0.15% of primary pleomorphic adenomas and 3.2% of recurrent pleomorphic adenomas.[15] Another more recent study suggested that in patients older than the age of 70, observation and upfront surgery have similar outcomes.[16] Thus, observation of pleomorphic adenoma may be warranted in select cases with the understanding of the real risk of malignant transformation.

DIAGNOSIS

Malignant tumors commonly present as a painless and palpable mass. Some signs that can help distinguish a malignant tumor from a benign neoplasm are rapid growth, pain, lymphadenopathy, and facial nerve weakness. Although facial nerve weakness or paralysis is highly indicative of a malignant mass, only about 20% of malignancies present with clinical facial nerve involvement.[17,18] Given the broad variety of clinical subtypes, pathologic diagnosis should be performed primarily through fine-needle aspiration cytology (FNAC).

Imaging

Imaging is not currently able to consistently distinguish between benign and malignant types of salivary tumors nor determine the specific subtype except by serial imaging. Ultrasound is used to localize the mass, identify pathologic cervical lymph nodes, and guide fine-needle aspiration.[19,20] The sonographic characteristics of heterogeneous echogenicity, poorly defined and irregular margins, local invasion, presence of calcifications, extraparenchymal extension, hypervascularity, and lack of deep enhancement more often indicate malignancy, but are not highly specific and do not provide clues for the histologic subtype of the tumor.[21,22]

MRI is the modality of choice for evaluating SGC especially for malignant tumors. MRI is superior for identifying tumor extent, invasion, and importantly the presence and degree of macroscopic perineural spread.[19] Similarly to ultrasound, there are findings that can point to malignancy, namely, irregular margins, heterogeneous masses, local invasion, hypointense lesions on T2-weighted imaging, and pathologic-appearing lymph nodes. However, similarly to ultrasound imaging, these findings are not always present, especially in early stage malignancy. Although MRI findings do not predict the underlying histology of the disease,[23] techniques using quantitative dynamic contrast-enhanced MRI and diffusion-weighted MRI have been shown to detect malignant versus benign salivary disease[24] and possibly even distinguish certain histologic subtypes.[25,26]

Computed tomography (CT) is less sensitive and specific than MRI in the evaluation of salivary gland disease[27] especially in identifying nerve involvement or extent of the lesion, but should be considered when MRI is not available or otherwise contraindicated. Combined 18F-fluorodeoxyglucose PET/CT is less helpful than in other forms of head and neck cancer. PET/CT is useful in determining local tumor extent, nodal involvement, and importantly distant metastases, especially in high-grade malignancies.[28,29] PET/CT has a higher specificity, but a lower sensitivity in the localization of SGC when compared with squamous cell carcinoma,[30] which can lead to higher false-negative rates, especially in small or low-grade tumors. The other major issue with using PET/CT to diagnose malignant versus benign disease is benign tumors, such as pleomorphic adenoma and Warthin tumor, also demonstrate high uptake.[31]

Fine-Needle Aspiration

Given the difficulties with imaging characteristics of salivary gland neoplasms, the diagnosis of malignancy still hinges on a cytologic and ultimately a histologic diagnosis. Additionally, given the varying natural history of the malignant subtypes, different surgical approaches may be required. Thus, accurate cytologic diagnosis before surgical excision remains important. For tumors within the sublingual and minor salivary glands in the oral cavity, one can consider open surgical biopsy. For tumors of the parotid gland, this approach is not recommended given the possibility of seeding the tumor and injury risk to the facial nerve. Therefore, for neoplasms of the parotid glands, and the submandibular glands, FNAC, frequently with ultrasound guidance, is the recommended strategy.[32]

Unfortunately, FNAC is not without its difficulties and limitations. Current studies of the accuracy of FNAC show such high levels of heterogeneity that no definitive guidelines on its use have been made.[33] The pitfalls of FNAC include: the high number and diversity of subtypes, the low incidence of rare subtypes, complex morphology, and morphologic overlap between subtypes. Finally, for some subtypes, the diagnosis of malignancy is made based on tumor invasion, not cellular atypia, which cannot be assessed with cytologic samples alone.[34]

Prior studies have shown a discordance between FNAC results and final pathologic diagnosis to be 20% to 40%.[35] A systematic review of 64 studies found the sensitivity of FNAC for diagnosis of malignancy to be 76% and the specificity to be 97%.[33] Moreover, given the high level of diversity of histologic subtypes and low incidence of disease, low-volume treatment facilities are likely to have limited expertise in the pathologic diagnosis of these malignancies. In fact, the ability to predict grade based on FNAC has been shown to vary across institutions.[34] However, despite these roadblocks, FNAC is commonly used in presurgical diagnosis given its relative safety, ease of scheduling, lack of need for general anesthesia, and minimal to no risk of tumor seeding when compared with open excisional biopsy.[36]

Intraoperative frozen section analysis has become less common as FNAC has increased in popularity. Although some studies show frozen section analysis to be superior to FNAC,[37] others have found FNAC to be more accurate.[38] Intraoperative frozen section analysis still has clinical utility in determining extent of spread of malignancy intraoperatively, identifying tumor extent, and diagnosing malignancy when FNAC is nondiagnostic or does not correlate with intraoperative findings.

MANAGEMENT
Surgery

Upfront surgery consisting of complete tumor excision with clear margins is currently the primary management strategy for most SGCs. In an analysis of primary radiotherapy versus upfront surgery with adjuvant radiotherapy, the surgery-first group had better disease-specific survival and overall survival.[39] In a study of the National Cancer Institute's Surveillance, Epidemiology, and End Results Database, assessing more than 5000 patients with minor SGC, the hazard ratio for death among patients treated with surgery versus patients receiving other treatments was 0.55.[39,40]

For management of malignancies of the submandibular gland, the general strategy is for en bloc resection of the gland. If overlying skin, muscle, or nerves are involved they are generally also resected. The surgeon should be aware of the proximity of the marginal branch of the facial nerve superficial to the gland and the hypoglossal and lingual nerves, which are deep to the gland. Preservation of these nerves if they are uninvaded by cancer is paramount.

For oncologic surgeries of the sublingual gland, resection requires removal of the sublingual gland and debatably sometimes soft tissue of the floor of mouth and even the submandibular duct glands. As such the marginal branch of facial, hypoglossal, and lingual nerves are in close proximity. Resection of the lingual nerve is more likely in these cases because of its proximity to the sublingual gland and depending on the tumor, mandibular resection may also be necessary.[41]

Parotid tumors are managed most commonly with superficial parotidectomy with preservation of the branches of the facial nerve. Many surgeons manage benign lesions with an enucleation of the tumor without (or minimal) identification of the facial nerve. However, this strategy is most appropriate for smaller superficial lobe tumors that do not grossly involve the facial nerve. Although enucleation offers the advantage of a limited incision and potentially lower rates of postoperative complications compared with more extensive procedures, such as superficial or total parotidectomy, it is not without problems. The risk of tumor recurrence must be carefully weighed against the benefits of gland preservation, particularly in cases where the tumor demonstrates aggressive features or histologic uncertainty.[42] If the tumor is in the deep lobe of the parotid or extends into the parapharyngeal space then total parotidectomy with parapharyngeal space dissection is the approach.

Management of surgical margins

Although postoperative radiation is widely accepted as standard of care for high-grade SGC, postoperative management of low- and intermediate-grade salivary carcinomas has been a topic of research. Margins used in the surgical resection of these tumors require weighing the risks and benefits of functional losses including but not limited to tumor proximity to the facial nerve for parotid tumors. Additionally, the effect of postoperative radiation on salivary function and associated quality of life are important factors. In a 30-year review of SGC at Memorial Sloan Kettering, Hanson and colleagues[43] found that close surgical margins (defined as <1 mm) for low- and intermediate-grade tumors were not risk factors for decreased disease-specific survival in patients who did not receive postoperative radiation compared with those who did. The American Head and Neck Society Salivary Gland Section, with a 10-year review across 41 institutions in five countries analyzing 865 patients,[44] evaluated the impact of radiation in patients with close margins in low- and intermediate-grade cancers. Most patients (93%) had parotid malignancy, and 86% were low grade, whereas 14% were intermediate grade; 35% underwent postoperative radiation and 79% had close margins (defined as ≤1 mm). No statistically significant difference was found for local recurrence for patients with close margins as their sole potential risk factors whether they underwent radiation (0%) or observation (2%) with a median (interquartile range) follow-up of 38.2 months (20.7–57.9). The 3-year local recurrence-free survival for the close margin group was 97%, comparable with the 96% survival of the overall study population highlighting that individuals with close margins likely can be observed safely.

Surgical approach

There are several unique aesthetic considerations when surgically managing parotid neoplasms. The first consideration is the type of incision. Generally, two types of incisions are commonly used: the modified facelift incision and the modified Blair incision. The modified facelift incision tends to be more appropriate for smaller (<3 cm) tumors that are posteriorly based in the lower two-thirds of the parotid. These two approaches have similar complication rates (seroma, hematoma, flap loss, facial nerve paralysis), but the facelift incision approach has been shown to lead to better patient-reported cosmetic outcomes.[45]

Another aesthetic and functional consideration is the management of the facial nerve. If the facial nerve is not invaded by malignant tumor, the goal of the surgeon is to identify and preserve the branches of the nerve. The use of intraoperative nerve monitoring has been shown to reduce the rate and duration of temporary facial nerve paralysis in parotid surgery,[46,47] especially revision surgery. However, a recent meta-analysis of studies report this correlation to be weak and suggest additional prospective, randomized trials.[48] Overall, the rate of permanent nerve paralysis after conservative parotidectomy is reported to be less than 5%.[47] The reported rate of temporary palsy is highly variable and reported between 15% and 65%.[49] Patients who present with facial nerve weakness have a significantly worse prognosis compared with patients with normal facial nerve functioning at diagnosis.[50]

There is not clear consensus about proper management of the preoperatively functional facial nerve in parotid malignancies. During some operations, the facial nerve may be found to be obviously adherent to, surrounded by, and/or invaded by tumor. In these situations, a decision needs to be made to either sacrifice the nerve or to dissect the tumor and preserve the facial nerve structure. Some studies do support preserving the facial nerve with microscopic residual disease on the nerve sheath when postoperative radiation is possible.[47,51,52] Newer research on management of the facial nerve has shown that up to 30% of patients who present with preoperative weakness can show no gross involvement of the facial nerve during surgical resection.[52] Although these authors report on a small number of patients (n = 45), they found similar oncologic outcomes in those with facial nerve sacrifice compared with those where the facial nerve was spared if there was no evidence of gross tumor involvement.[52] In cases where the margins are close to the nerve, some recommend preservation and suggest that local adjuvant radiotherapy can improve local control of disease.[53,54]

Other studies show possibly better oncologic outcomes with facial nerve sacrifice.[55] Studies have shown that in ACC facial nerve sacrifice should be performed if needed to obtain clear surgical margins because this leads to improved local control and overall survival.[55,56] However, patients with facial nerve sacrifice reported significantly lower quality of life.[55]

With parotidectomy surgery, the surgeon should consider the restoration of the contour defect associated with the ablation. Free abdominal fat graft transfer has been shown to be a safe and effective way for restoring contour in parotidectomy defects.[57,58] There may be some degree of atrophy of the fat; thus, a 30% overcorrection of the graft harvest can be performed to compensate for this expected volume loss. A variety of local flaps have also been described in the closure of parotidectomy defects including: sternocleidomastoid advancement flaps, temporoparietal fascial flaps, superficial musculoaponeurotic system flaps or superficial musculoaponeurotic system plications, and acellular matrix grafts.[59,60] These local reconstruction options lead to improved aesthetic outcomes and patient satisfaction.[61–63] Additionally, free fat transfer and local advancement flaps have been shown to significantly decrease the rate of Frey syndrome postoperatively.[64] Theoretically the graft blocks the extension of free parotid parasympathetic nerves to the overlying sweat glands.

For larger parotidectomy defects, a deepithelialized anterolateral thigh free flap has been described as a means to restore contour to the area.[65] Anterolateral thigh flaps are considered potentially important to consider when a patient is planning for postoperative radiation therapy to maintain contour. Deepithelialized anterolateral thigh free flaps in the parotid have been shown to maintain a stable size, even after radiotherapy,[66] with as low as 8% fat loss.[67] This makes them a potentially more stable construct than the free abdominal fat transfer.

Neck dissection

Cervical nodal metastases are a well-known negative prognostic factor for SGC.[68,69] Factors that increase the risk of cervical nodal disease include tumor size,[69,70] histologic subtype,[69,71] and tumor grade.[72] In a clinically or radiologically positive neck, the current recommendation for a therapeutic neck dissection includes level I to IV and possibly V.

The surgical management of the clinically node-negative neck is more controversial. Meta analysis of 22 studies shows that the overall occult nodal metastasis rate in SGC is 21%. This proportion was significantly higher in T3/T4 disease (36%) and in tumors with high-grade histology (34%).[73] These authors recommend elective neck dissection of levels II to III in patients with T3/T4 tumors or tumors of unknown or high-grade histology in the parotid gland. They also recommend the addition of level I in submandibular, sublingual, and minor salivary glands that meet these criteria. However, there are no definitive recommendations for which levels to include in the dissection, because the levels of dissection included do not show definitive improvement in recurrence or survival rates.[74] We recommend the inclusion of levels 1b, 2a, 2b, and 3. We believe that this approach leads to more accurate staging and helps target the radiation dose or can eliminate the needs for adjuvant radiation in certain cases. The morbidity of a 1b to 3 elective neck dissection is rarely very negatively impactful in experienced surgeon's hangs.

The intraoperative sequence of the neck dissection being performed before a parotidectomy can facilitate resection of the primary tumor. In these authors' opinion, performing the neck dissection before the parotidectomy can limit the early exposure of the facial nerve, and improve exposure of the inferior portion of the parotid gland and the marginal mandibular nerve.

Radiation

Although upfront surgery leads to a better survival than primary radiation, adjuvant radiation does have a role for high-grade and some advanced-stage SGC. Low-grade SGC can generally be observed after adequate surgical resection. Postoperative adjuvant radiotherapy has been shown to be an independent positive factor for overall survival in patients with high-grade SGC.[75,76] Currently, adjuvant radiotherapy is recommended in undifferentiated or high-grade tumors, tumors with perineural invasion, tumors with advanced disease including facial nerve involvement or deep parotid lobe involvement, and all ACCs.[77,78] Definitive radiation therapy can also be considered in inoperable tumors or in patients who are unable to undergo surgery.

Adjuvant radiation can also be considered for the management of the clinically negative neck. In a study of 251 SGCs treated with surgery and primary site radiation, the addition of elective neck radiation decreased the nodal relapse rate from 26% to 0%.[79] The authors of this study recommend the use of elective neck radiation in select patients with high risk of regional failure. Another study of patients with clinically node-negative disease with high-grade histology underwent either elective neck dissection and radiation or just elective neck irradiation. The rate of occult metastases in the elective neck dissection group was about 40%. However, there was no additional cause-specific increase in survival for patients who underwent neck dissection and neck irradiation.[80] Therefore, these authors argue that either elective neck dissection or elective neck radiation leads to improved locoregional control. Current recommendations for the N0 neck are to consider elective neck dissection and/or elective radiation in high-grade tumors, T3/T4 tumors, primary tumors greater than 3 cm, involvement of the facial nerve, extraglandular tumor spread, patients with age greater than 54, and the presence of perineural invasion.[74]

Systemic Therapy

The addition of chemotherapy to adjuvant radiation therapy for SGC has not been shown to increase overall survival.[81] In some studies, it has actually been shown to increase overall mortality and toxicity among patients.[82] RTOG-1008 (NCT01220583) is an ongoing clinical trial analyzing progressive-free survival in patients with high-risk SGC who are randomized to adjuvant radiation or chemoradiation with cisplatin postoperatively.

The specific mutational burden of SGC provides potential targets for systemic therapy and remains an area of investigation. Up to 90% of patients with salivary ductal carcinoma carry androgen receptor positivity, whereas 30% to 40% are positive for human epidermal growth factor receptor 2 (HER2).[83] HER-2 antagonists, such as trastuzumab, and antibody drug conjugates specific for HER2 are highly effective (eg, trastuzumab deruxtecan [Enhertu]) are emerging options for salivary ductal carcinoma.[83] Tyrosine kinase inhibitors (TKI) including vascular endothelial growth factor receptor inhibitors, such as lenvatinib and axitinib, are less promising areas of active study for advanced and metastatic SGC.[84]

Treatment of Distant Metastases in Adenoid Cystic Carcinoma

A defining feature of ACC is its metastatic potential with metastases or recurrence occurring in approximately 30% to 40% of patients in the 10 to 15 years posttreatment, most commonly to the lungs.[50,85] Of those with lung metastases, up to 95% of patients have no symptoms at time of diagnosis.[86] Additionally, data demonstrate that mean survival following detection of lung metastases is approximately 4 years compared with 19 to 21 months for bony metastases.[84]

At present, there are no Food and Drug Administration–approved systemic therapies for distant metastases in SGC including high-risk ACC. Current data suggest that individuals with oligometastases can be treated with surgery or radiation. Given slow progression of metastatic disease in lungs, they can also be observed. However, for rapidly growing or symptomatic metastatic disease, patients may be amenable to systemic treatment with TKI, traditional chemotherapy, or considered for the RTOG-1008 trial.[84] Vascular endothelial growth factor receptor inhibitors belonging to the family of TKI including lenvatinib and axitinib have emerged as potential treatment options in phase II clinical trials demonstrating modest improvement in progression-free survival.[84] Platinum-based chemotherapy may also be used but has demonstrated minimal benefit in prior studies with a much higher cytotoxic profile.

SURVEILLANCE

Rates of locoregional recurrence can vary greatly among subtypes of SGC with it generally being very low for low-grade SGC and higher for high-grade cancers. Five-year local recurrence rates in ACC have been reported to be 40%, whereas the rate of distant metastases ranges between 8% and 60%.[50] However, the local rates of recurrence for mucoepidermoid carcinoma have been reported to be around 4%, with rates of distant metastases around 12%.[87] The National Comprehensive Cancer Network guidelines currently recommend surveillance of SGC to follow similar protocols as that of other cancers of the upper aerodigestive tract.[88] These guidelines recommend patients begin with quarterly surveillance, consisting of the patient's history and physical examination for the first 2 to 3 years posttreatment. These can be spaced to biannual visits until 5 years posttreatment, and then spaced to yearly visits indefinitely.[89] This is recommended because a significant portion of patients who are clear of disease at 5-year follow-up have been shown to develop late recurrences.[90]

Regarding posttreatment surveillance imaging the American Society of Clinical Oncology recommends baseline imaging to be completed 3 months after treatment with a contrast MRI. PET/CT can also be obtained if clinically available and CT with contrast is considered if patients are unable to perform MRI. After that, contrast CT or MRI is obtained every 6 to 12 months for the next 2 years posttreatment. They also recommend contrast CT of the chest. From posttreatment years 3 to 5, imaging is offered based on clinical concern or yearly for patients with high-grade histology or poor prognostic factors. After 5 years, yearly chest CT is offered to patients with ACC, high-grade histology, or other poor prognostic factors.[91] Chest imaging is recommended, because the lungs are the most common site of distant metastasis (particularly for ACC), and this risk is higher in high-grade histologic subtypes.[92]

SUMMARY

SGC is made up of a large variety of histologic subtypes that affect the parotid, submandibular, sublingual, and minor salivary glands. The different subtypes have a different clinical course, which can affect management decisions. Obtaining an accurate histologic diagnosis before surgical resection remains challenging and although FNAC is helpful, it is often unable to provide specific diagnostic information. Although it is agreed that upfront surgery for the primary site and clinically evident cervical nodal metastasis is critical for improvement in survival, there is still debate about the management of the clinically node-negative neck. The rate of occult cervical metastases in certain histologic subtypes is high and elective neck dissection and elective neck radiation seem to improve survival. Chemotherapy does not seem to improve the overall survival in SGC, but may have a role in the management of distant metastatic disease. Posttreatment surveillance of these patients is important, because many histologic subtypes can present with late local recurrence and distant metastases many years after apparently successful treatment.

CLINICS CARE POINTS

- Based on the most recent World Health Organization classification there are 21 different subtypes of malignant and 15 subtypes of benign salivary gland tumors.

- The most common SGC are mucoepidermoid and adenoid cystic carcinoma. Squamous cell carcinoma is also common in salivary glands, but its presence usually indicates a cutaneous metastasis rather than a primary tumor.

- Malignancies present as a painless, enlarging mass. In the parotid gland they may also present with facial nerve weakness.

- MRI is the preoperative imaging modality of choice because it is the best modality to determine perineural invasion.

- FNAC with or without ultrasound is commonly used to obtain a preoperative tissue diagnosis, but it is difficult to obtain a specific histologic diagnosis. Intraoperative frozen section are used to determine location of disease intraoperatively and when the preoperative diagnosis is unclear.

- Surgery is the modality of choice for primary tumors. In parotid malignancies, reconstruction of the defect improves patient cosmesis and decreases rates of postoperative Frey syndrome.

- In a clinically node-negative neck, the rate of clinically occult cervical nodes is 30% from subhistologic subtypes. For high-risk malignancies (high grade, T3/T4) elective neck dissection or elective neck radiation should be considered. There is a limited role for chemotherapy or immunotherapy in the primary treatment of SGC.

- Adenoid cystic carcinoma has a high rate of late metastatic recurrence, especially to the lungs.

• Posttreatment surveillance should be at least quarterly for the first 2 to 3 years, then spaced biannually until 5 years, and then spaced to yearly. CT chest should be performed yearly for those with adenoid cystic carcinoma.

DISCLOSURE

The authors have nothing to disclose.

REFERENCES

1. Boukheris H, Curtis RE, Land CE, et al. Incidence of carcinoma of the major salivary glands according to the WHO classification, 1992 to 2006: a population-based study in the United States. Cancer Epidemiol Biomarkers Prev 2009;18: 2899–906.
2. Carvalho AL, Nishimoto IN, Califano JA, et al. Trends in incidence and prognosis for head and neck cancer in the United States: a site-specific analysis of the SEER database. Int J Cancer 2005;114:806–16.
3. Thompson L. World Health Organization classification of tumours: pathology and genetics of head and neck tumours. Ear Nose Throat J 2006;85:74.
4. Skálová A, Hyrcza MD, Leivo I. Update from the 5th Edition of the world health organization classification of head and neck tumors: salivary glands. Head Neck Pathol 2022;16:40–53.
5. El-Naggar AK, Chan JKC, Grandis JR, et al. WHO classification of head and neck tumours. International Agency for Research on Cancer; 2017.
6. Kakarala K, Bhattacharyya N. Survival in oral cavity minor salivary gland carcinoma. Otolaryngol Head Neck Surg 2010;143:122–6.
7. Eveson JW, Cawson RA. Salivary gland tumours. A review of 2410 cases with particular reference to histological types, site, age and sex distribution. J Pathol 1985;146:51–8.
8. Bjørndal K, Krogdahl A, Therkildsen MH, et al. Salivary gland carcinoma in Denmark 1990-2005: a national study of incidence, site and histology. Results of the Danish Head and Neck Cancer Group (DAHANCA). Oral Oncol 2011;47: 677–82.
9. Spiro RH. Salivary neoplasms: overview of a 35-year experience with 2,807 patients. Head Neck Surg 1986;8:177–84.
10. Boukheris H, Ron E, Dores GM, et al. Risk of radiation-related salivary gland carcinomas among survivors of Hodgkin lymphoma: a population-based analysis. Cancer 2008;113:3153–9.
11. Sadetzki S, Oberman B, Mandelzweig L, et al. Smoking and risk of parotid gland tumors: a nationwide case-control study. Cancer 2008;112:1974–82.
12. Eneroth CM, Zetterberg A. Malignancy in pleomorphic adenoma. A clinical and microspectrophotometric study. Acta Otolaryngol 1974;77:426–32.
13. Zhan KY, Khaja SF, Flack AB, et al. Benign parotid tumors. Otolaryngol. Clin. North Am 2016;49:327–42.
14. Andreasen S, Therkildsen MH, Bjørndal K, et al. Pleomorphic adenoma of the parotid gland 1985-2010: a Danish nationwide study of incidence, recurrence rate, and malignant transformation. Head Neck 2016;38(Suppl 1):E1364–9.
15. Valstar MH, de Ridder M, van den Broek EC, et al. Salivary gland pleomorphic adenoma in the Netherlands: a nationwide observational study of primary tumor incidence, malignant transformation, recurrence, and risk factors for recurrence. Oral Oncol 2017;66:93–9.

16. Kligerman MP, Jin M, Ayoub N, et al. Comparison of parotidectomy with observation for treatment of pleomorphic adenoma in adults. JAMA Otolaryngol. Head Neck Surg 2020;146:1027–34.
17. Terhaard C, Lubsen H, Tan B, et al. Facial nerve function in carcinoma of the parotid gland. Eur J Cancer 2006;42:2744–50.
18. Eneroth CM. Facial nerve paralysis. a criterion of malignancy in parotid tumors. Arch Otolaryngol 1972;95:300–4.
19. Lee YYP, Wong KT, King AD, et al. Imaging of salivary gland tumours. Eur J Radiol 2008;66:419–36.
20. Gritzmann N, Rettenbacher T, Hollerweger A, et al. Sonography of the salivary glands. Eur Radiol 2003;13:964–75.
21. Kovacević DO, Fabijanić I. Sonographic diagnosis of parotid gland lesions: correlation with the results of sonographically guided fine-needle aspiration biopsy. J Clin Ultrasound 2010;38:294–8.
22. Zheng M, Plonowska KA, Strohl MP, et al. Surgeon-performed ultrasound for the assessment of parotid masses. Am J Otolaryngol 2018;39:467–71.
23. Freling NJ, Molenaar WM, Vermey A, et al. Malignant parotid tumors: clinical use of MR imaging and histologic correlation. Radiology 1992;185:691–6.
24. Yabuuchi H, Fukuya T, Tajima T, et al. Salivary gland tumors: diagnostic value of gadolinium-enhanced dynamic MR imaging with histopathologic correlation. Radiology 2003;226:345–54.
25. Habermann CR, Arndt C, Graessner J, et al. Diffusion-weighted echo-planar MR imaging of primary parotid gland tumors: is a prediction of different histologic subtypes possible? AJNR Am. J. Neuroradiol 2009;30:591–6.
26. Rodriguez JD, Selleck AM, Abdel Razek AAK, et al. Update on MR imaging of soft tissue tumors of head and neck. Magn. Reson. Imaging Clin. N. Am 2022; 30:151–98.
27. Hanna E, Vural E, Prokopakis E, et al. The sensitivity and specificity of high-resolution imaging in evaluating perineural spread of adenoid cystic carcinoma to the skull base. Arch Otolaryngol Head Neck Surg 2007;133:541–5.
28. Roh J-L, Ryu CH, Choi SH, et al. Clinical utility of 18F-FDG PET for patients with salivary gland malignancies. J Nucl Med 2007;48:240–6.
29. Jeong H-S, Chung MK, Son YI, et al. Role of 18F-FDG PET/CT in management of high-grade salivary gland malignancies. J Nucl Med 2007;48:1237–44.
30. Branstetter BF, Blodgett TM, Zimmer LA, et al. 4thHead and neck malignancy: is PET/CT more accurate than PET or CT alone? Radiology 2005;235:580–6.
31. Keyes JW, Harkness BA, Greven KM, et al. Salivary gland tumors: pretherapy evaluation with PET. Radiology 1994;192:99–102.
32. Kechagias N, Ntomouchtsis A, Valeri R, et al. Fine-needle aspiration cytology of salivary gland tumours: a 10-year retrospective analysis. Oral Maxillofac. Surg 2012;16:35–40.
33. Schmidt RL, Hall BJ, Wilson AR, et al. A systematic review and meta-analysis of the diagnostic accuracy of fine-needle aspiration cytology for parotid gland lesions. Am J Clin Pathol 2011;136:45–59.
34. Westra WH. Diagnostic difficulties in the classification and grading of salivary gland tumors. Int J Radiat Oncol Biol Phys 2007;69:S49–51.
35. Colella G, Cannavale R, Flamminio F, et al. Fine-needle aspiration cytology of salivary gland lesions: a systematic review. J Oral Maxillofac Surg 2010;68:2146–53.
36. Shah KSV, Ethunandan M. Tumour seeding after fine-needle aspiration and core biopsy of the head and neck: a systematic review. Br J Oral Maxillofac Surg 2016; 54:260–5.

37. Zbären P, Nuyens M, Loosli H, et al. Diagnostic accuracy of fine-needle aspiration cytology and frozen section in primary parotid carcinoma. Cancer 2004;100: 1876–83.
38. Seethala RR, LiVolsi VA, Baloch ZW. Relative accuracy of fine-needle aspiration and frozen section in the diagnosis of lesions of the parotid gland. Head Neck 2005;27:217–23.
39. Holtzman A, Morris CG, Amdur RJ, et al. Outcomes after primary or adjuvant radiotherapy for salivary gland carcinoma. Acta Oncol 2017;56:484–9.
40. Baddour HM Jr, Fedewa SA, Chen AY. Five- and 10-year cause-specific survival rates in carcinoma of the minor salivary gland. JAMA Otolaryngol. Head Neck Surg 2016;142:67–73.
41. Rinaldo A, Shaha AR, Pellitteri PK, et al. Management of malignant sublingual salivary gland tumors. Oral Oncol 2004;40:2–5.
42. Taguchi A, Kojima T, Okanoue Y, et al. Validation of indications for enucleation for benign parotid gland tumors. Head Neck 2023;45(4):931–8.
43. Hanson M, et al. Evaluation of surgical margin status in patients with salivary gland cancer. JAMA Otolaryngol. Head Neck Surg 2022;148:128–38.
44. Sajisevi M, et al. Oncologic safety of close margins in patients with low- to intermediate-grade major salivary gland carcinoma. JAMA otolaryngology–head & neck surgery 2024;150:107–16.
45. Grover N, D'Souza A. Facelift approach for parotidectomy: an evolving aesthetic technique. Otolaryngol Head Neck Surg 2013;148:548–56.
46. Eisele DW, Wang SJ, Orloff LA. Electrophysiologic facial nerve monitoring during parotidectomy. Head Neck 2010;32:399–405.
47. Guntinas-Lichius O, et al. Primary parotid malignoma surgery in patients with normal preoperative facial nerve function: outcome and long-term postoperative facial nerve function. Laryngoscope 2004;114:949–56.
48. Chiesa-Estomba CM, et al. Facial nerve monitoring during parotid gland surgery: a systematic review and meta-analysis. Eur Arch Oto-Rhino-Laryngol 2021;278: 933–43.
49. Siddiqui AH, Shakil S, Rahim DU, et al. Post parotidectomy facial nerve palsy: a retrospective analysis. Pak J Med Sci Q 2020;36:126–30.
50. Terhaard CHJ, et al. Salivary gland carcinoma: independent prognostic factors for locoregional control, distant metastases, and overall survival: results of the Dutch head and neck oncology cooperative group. Head Neck 2004;26: 681–92, discussion 692–3.
51. Iyer NG, Clark JR, Murali R, et al. Outcomes following parotidectomy for metastatic squamous cell carcinoma with microscopic residual disease: implications for facial nerve preservation. Head Neck 2009;31:21–7.
52. Park W, et al. Clinical outcomes and management of facial nerve in patients with parotid gland cancer and pretreatment facial weakness. Oral Oncol 2019;89: 144–9.
53. Spiro JD, Spiro RH. Cancer of the parotid gland: role of 7th nerve preservation. World J Surg 2003;27:863–7.
54. El-Shakhs S, Khalil Y, Abdou AG. Facial nerve preservation in total parotidectomy for parotid tumors: a review of 27 cases. Ear Nose Throat J 2013;92:E1.
55. Iseli TA, et al. Facial nerve sacrifice and radiotherapy in parotid adenoid cystic carcinoma. Laryngoscope 2008;118:1781–6.
56. Casler JD, Conley JJ. Surgical management of adenoid cystic carcinoma in the parotid gland. Otolaryngol Head Neck Surg 1992;106:332–8.

57. Conger BT, Gourin CG. Free abdominal fat transfer for reconstruction of the total parotidectomy defect. Laryngoscope 2008;118:1186–90.
58. Loyo M, Gourin CG. Free abdominal fat transfer for partial and total parotidectomy defect reconstruction. Laryngoscope 2016;126:2694–8.
59. Tamplen M, Knott PD, Fritz MA, et al. Controversies in parotid defect reconstruction. Facial Plast Surg Clin. North Am 2016;24:235–43.
60. Militsakh ON, Sanderson JA, Lin D, et al. Rehabilitation of a parotidectomy patient: a systematic approach. Head Neck 2013;35:1349–61.
61. Chow TL, Lam CY, Chiu PW, et al. Sternomastoid-muscle transposition improves the cosmetic outcome of superficial parotidectomy. Br J Plast Surg 2001;54: 409–11.
62. Chen W, et al. SMAS fold flap and ADM repair of the parotid bed following removal of parotid haemangiomas via pre- and retroauricular incisions to improve cosmetic outcome and prevent Frey's syndrome. J Plast Reconstr Aesthet Surg 2008;61:894–9, discussion 899–900.
63. Mianroodi AA, et al. Autologous free dermal-fat-fascial graft for parotidectomy defects: a case series. Ann Otol Rhinol Laryngol 2021;130:1171–80.
64. Li C, Yang X, Pan J, et al. Graft for prevention of Frey syndrome after parotidectomy: a systematic review and meta-analysis of randomized controlled trials. J Oral Maxillofac Surg 2013;71:419–27.
65. Cannady SB, Seth R, Fritz MA, et al. Total parotidectomy defect reconstruction using the buried free flap. Otolaryngol Head Neck Surg 2010;143:637–43.
66. Strohl MP, et al. Long-term stability of vascularized adipofascial flaps in facial reconstruction. Facial Plast Surg Aesthet Med 2020;22:262–7.
67. Higgins KM, et al. Volumetric changes of the anterolateral thigh free flap following adjuvant radiotherapy in total parotidectomy reconstruction. Laryngoscope 2012; 122:767–72.
68. Bhattacharyya N, Fried MP. Nodal metastasis in major salivary gland cancer: predictive factors and effects on survival. Arch Otolaryngol Head Neck Surg 2002; 128:904–8.
69. Megwalu UC, Sirjani D. Risk of nodal metastasis in major salivary gland adenoid cystic carcinoma. Otolaryngol Head Neck Surg 2017;156:660–4.
70. Rodríguez-Cuevas S, Labastida S, Baena L, et al. Risk of nodal metastases from malignant salivary gland tumors related to tumor size and grade of malignancy. Eur Arch Oto-Rhino-Laryngol 1995;252:139–42.
71. Lloyd S, Yu JB, Ross DA, et al. A prognostic index for predicting lymph node metastasis in minor salivary gland cancer. Int J Radiat Oncol Biol Phys 2010; 76:169–75.
72. Ellis MA, Graboyes EM, Day TA, et al. Prognostic factors and occult nodal disease in mucoepidermoid carcinoma of the oral cavity and oropharynx: an analysis of the National Cancer Database. Oral Oncol 2017;72:174–8.
73. Westergaard-Nielsen M, et al. Elective neck dissection in patients with salivary gland carcinoma: a systematic review and meta-analysis. J Oral Pathol Med 2020;49:606–16.
74. Spiegel JH, Jalisi S. Contemporary diagnosis and management of head and neck cancer. Otolaryngol Clin North Am 2005;38:xiii–xiv.
75. Safdieh J, et al. Impact of adjuvant radiotherapy for malignant salivary gland tumors. Otolaryngol Head Neck Surg 2017;157:988–94.
76. Mahmood U, Koshy M, Goloubeva O, et al. Adjuvant radiation therapy for high-grade and/or locally advanced major salivary gland tumors. Arch Otolaryngol Head Neck Surg 2011;137:1025–30.

77. Terhaard CHJ, et al. The role of radiotherapy in the treatment of malignant salivary gland tumors. Int J Radiat Oncol Biol Phys 2005;61:103–11.
78. Chen AM, Garcia J, Granchi P, et al. Base of skull recurrences after treatment of salivary gland cancer with perineural invasion reduced by postoperative radiotherapy. Clin Otolaryngol 2009;34:539–45.
79. Chen AM, Garcia J, Lee NY, et al. Patterns of nodal relapse after surgery and postoperative radiation therapy for carcinomas of the major and minor salivary glands: what is the role of elective neck irradiation? Int J Radiat Oncol Biol Phys 2007;67:988–94.
80. Herman MP, et al. Elective neck management for high-grade salivary gland carcinoma. Am J Otolaryngol 2013;34:205–8.
81. Amini A, et al. Association of adjuvant chemoradiotherapy vs radiotherapy alone with survival in patients with resected major salivary gland carcinoma: data from the national cancer data base. JAMA Otolaryngol Head Neck Surg 2016;142:1100–10.
82. Tanvetyanon T, et al. Adjuvant chemoradiotherapy versus with radiotherapy alone for locally advanced salivary gland carcinoma among older patients. Head Neck 2016;38:863–70.
83. Takahashi H, et al. Phase II trial of trastuzumab and docetaxel in patients with human epidermal growth factor receptor 2-positive salivary duct carcinoma. J Clin Oncol 2019;37:125–34.
84. Lee RH, Wai KC, Chan JW, et al. Approaches to the management of metastatic adenoid cystic carcinoma. Cancers 2022;14.
85. Spiro RH. Distant metastasis in adenoid cystic carcinoma of salivary origin. Am J Surg 1997;174:495–8.
86. Sung M-W, et al. Clinicopathologic predictors and impact of distant metastasis from adenoid cystic carcinoma of the head and neck. Arch Otolaryngol Head Neck Surg 2003;129:1193–7.
87. Singareddy R, et al. Mucoepidermoid carcinoma of the salivary gland: long term outcomes from a tertiary cancer center in India. Indian J Otolaryngol Head Neck Surg 2022;74:1763–7.
88. Pfister DG, et al. Head and neck cancers, version 2.2020, NCCN clinical practice guidelines in oncology. J Natl Compr Cancer Netw 2020;18:873–98.
89. Digonnet A, et al. Follow-up strategies in head and neck cancer other than upper aerodigestive tract squamous cell carcinoma. Eur Arch Oto-Rhino-Laryngol 2013;270:1981–9.
90. Chen AM, Garcia J, Granchi PJ, et al. Late recurrence from salivary gland cancer: when does 'cure' mean cure? Cancer 2008;112:340–4.
91. Geiger JL, et al. Management of salivary gland malignancy: ASCO guideline. J Clin Oncol 2021;39:1909–41.
92. Ali S, et al. Distant metastases in patients with carcinoma of the major salivary glands. Ann Surg Oncol 2015;22:4014–9.

Laryngeal Preservation Strategies

Tam Ramsey, MD[a,1], Raisa Tikhtman, MD[a,2], Alice L. Tang, MD[a,*]

KEYWORDS

- Laryngeal preservation surgery • Laryngeal cancer • Conservation laryngeal surgery
- Laryngeal management

KEY POINTS

- For treatment of early laryngeal cancer, the preferred approach involves a single modality, either radiation or surgery, to minimize side effects of bimodality treatment.
- In cases of advanced stage cancer, the current recommendation is a combination of treatments, such as surgery with adjuvant radiation/chemoradiation or concurrent chemoradiation.
- Total laryngectomy followed by postoperative radiation is strongly considered for patients with tracheostomy tube dependence, severe dysphagia, and thyroid cartilage involvement.
- Endoscopic resection is preferred over open partial laryngectomy in early-stage laryngeal cancers.
- Supracricoid laryngectomy is recognized as a valuable alternative to total laryngectomy in select cases, including salvage resection.

INTRODUCTION

According to the National Cancer Institute, laryngeal cancer will affect approximately 12,380 patients and inflict an estimated 3820 deaths in 2023.[1] The most established risk factors for laryngeal cancer are tobacco and alcohol use that are synergistic and account for 89% of laryngeal cancers.[2] Improved awareness of tobacco and alcohol as leading etiologies has led to a slight decline in incidence at a rate of 2.4% yearly.[1] The role of human papillomavirus (HPV) in laryngeal cancer has remained controversial and is not currently employed in staging and prognostic evaluations as with oropharyngeal cancer.[3,4] The overall 5 year survival rate for laryngeal cancer stands at 61.6% between 2013 and 2019, without an appreciable change compared to 60.7% in the 5 years prior.[1,5,6]

[a] Department of Otolaryngology–Head & Neck Surgery, University of Cincinnati, College of Medicine, 3151 Bellevue Avenue, Cincinnati, OH 45219, USA
[1] Present address: 2533 Woodburn Avenue, Apartment 547B, Cincinnati, OH 45206.
[2] Present address: 453 Milton Street, Cincinnati, OH 45202.
* Corresponding author. 3151 Bellevue Avenue, Cincinnati, OH 45219.
E-mail address: alice.tang@uc.edu

Surg Oncol Clin N Am 33 (2024) 761–773
https://doi.org/10.1016/j.soc.2024.04.009
1055-3207/24/© 2024 Elsevier Inc. All rights reserved.

surgonc.theclinics.com

Surgery was the mainstay of treatment of laryngeal cancer before the availability of chemotherapy and radiation. The first laryngeal preservation surgery was a hemilaryngectomy performed by Billroth in 1874.[7] Since then, laryngeal surgery has fluctuated in popularity. Many have adopted the use of radiation alone for early-stage cancer and concurrent chemoradiation for late-stage laryngeal cancer in an attempt to conserve laryngeal function. For head and neck surgeons or general otolaryngologists who are unfamiliar with conservation laryngeal surgeries (CLS), the nonsurgical options are appealing. This article will review the current recommendations and different surgical options for laryngeal cancer.

LARYNGEAL ANATOMY

Understanding the function and anatomy of the larynx is paramount when treating patients with laryngeal cancer. The principal functions of the larynx are airway protection, phonation, and swallowing. These essential functions hinge on intricate coordination of the cricoarytenoid units, each comprised an arytenoid, the cricoid cartilage, interarytenoid muscles, ipsilateral posterior cricoarytenoid muscle, lateral cricoarytenoid muscle, and the superior and recurrent laryngeal nerves. The unit is responsible for laryngeal function and at least 1 of the 2 units should remain intact in CLS. Arytenoid fixation, as opposed to vocal cord immobility from tumor bulk, is a contraindication to CLS. Accordingly, preoperative workup should include an evaluation of the extent of the cancer and the probability of preserving the functional unit. The T stage in laryngeal cancer helps determine the prognosis and treatment options; however, it neither specifies the laryngeal structures involved nor specifies the type of CLS that may be performed. For example, a T2 glottic cancer with supraglottic spread may be amenable to CLS while a T2 glottic cancer with more than 1 cm extension into the subglottis is no longer a candidate for CLS.

Similarly, surgeons should possess an impeccable knowledge of laryngeal anatomy and the routes of or barriers to tumor spread. The anterior commissure consists of dense fibrous attachments between the vocal cords and thyroid cartilage, and it is devoid of perichondrium. In early-stage cancer, the anterior commissure functions as a barrier to spread, but in late-stage cancer, it may be a conduit for direct tumor extension to the thyroid cartilage.[8,9] Bagatella and colleagues demonstrated that supraglottic cancer spread tends to halt at the fibrous connective tissue above the anterior commissure.[10] Once it spreads to the glottis, supraglottic cancer is more likely to invade cartilage. Conversely, glottic cancer involving the anterior commissure tends to spread mucosally from one side to the other. Ulusan and colleagues confirmed this finding in his study of 62 patients undergoing supracricoid partial laryngectomy (SCPL). The rate of cartilage invasion was much lower in patients with glottic cancer involving the anterior commissure (5.4%) than in patients with supraglottic cancer involving the anterior commissure (32%).[11] Therefore, it is reasonable to perform endoscopic resection for the former while using open approaches for the latter.

The quadrangular membrane functions as a crucial impediment to the spread of supraglottic cancer into the glottis. Hajek and colleagues and then later Pressman and colleagues performed submucosal injections of the larynx that demonstrated a sharp demarcation of the inferior false cords and ventricles.[12,13] This illustrated the quadrangular membrane's efficacy as a barrier, with a clear boundary between supraglottic and glottic regions. Similarly, the conus elasticus and vocal ligament mitigate the local spread of early glottic carcinoma. However, it is noteworthy that, in advanced stages of cancer, the conus elasticus may serve as a conduit for the extension of glottic cancer into the subglottis. Additionally, surgeons should be aware of another elastic fibrous layer connecting the quadrangular and conus elasticus membranes that may facilitate supraglottic to glottic spread without apparent involvement of ventricular mucosa. This complex anatomy underscores the intricacies that surgeons must navigate in laryngeal surgeries.

Once a tumor invades the perichondrium, it may spread freely throughout the thyroid cartilage; thus, trans-thyroid cartilage resection in some CLS is not acceptable. It is difficult to identify cartilaginous invasion and even penetration of cancer through imaging. Fifty percentage of clinical T3 laryngeal cancers display only microinvasion of the thyroid cartilage on histologic examination.[14] Thyroid cartilage involvement should be suspected in cases with extensive cartilage ossification, glottic fixation, transglottic spread, and extensive involvement of the anterior commissure.[14]

The hyoid bone is rarely involved in laryngeal carcinoma; hyoid infiltration is mostly associated with vallecular involvement. Only 1.46% of 755 laryngectomy specimens for laryngeal cancer demonstrated hyoid invasion in one study.[15] Therefore, the hyoid should be spared for functional preservation if tumor does not involve vallecula. The hyoepiglottic ligament is a barrier of tumor spread from preepiglottic and paraglottic spaces to the vallecula and tongue base.[16] Serial sectioning through supraglottic cancer laryngectomy specimens revealed that infrahyoid laryngeal cancer did not spread beyond the hyoepiglottic ligament (**Fig. 1**). Tumors of the infrahyoid epiglottis enter the preepiglottic space through fenestrations in the epiglottic cartilage; the perichondrium forms a pseudocapsule around the tumor, and there is a lack of hyoid involvement. Therefore, tumors confined to the infrahyoid larynx do not need tongue base resection for margin.[9]

Tumors originated at the lingual epiglottis or vallecula may spread to the tongue base but are unlikely to invade the paraglottic and preglottic spaces due to

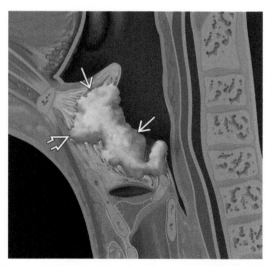

Fig. 1. An infrahyoid supraglottic tumor invading the preepiglottic space. Its extension is limited superiorly by hyoepiglottic ligament, sagittal view. (*Arrow*) outlines of a T3 supraglottic tumor. (*Arrow head*) tumor invasion of the preepiglottic space, abutting the thyrohyoid ligament. (*From* Gurgel RK, Harnsberger HR. Staging: Larynx. In: Harnsberger HR, ed. Imaging in Otolaryngology. Elsevier; [2018]:240-244.)

impedance from the hyoepiglottic ligament. Thus, limited supraglottic resection may be adequate. In contrast, suprahyoid laryngeal epiglottic cancers likely destroy the epiglottic cartilage and insertion of the hyoepiglotic ligament, thereby, facilitating invasion of the preglottic and paraglottic spaces with an easy access to the tongue base (**Fig. 2**).[17] Invasion of the oropharynx is also possible for aryepiglottic fold tumors, as the aryepiglottic fold confluences with the pharyngoepiglottic fold superiorly (note: the pharyngoepiglottic fold is the lateral border of the hyoepiglottic ligament).

PRETREATMENT WORKUP

A thorough history and physical examination should be done to assess the functional impairment and the extent of the cancer. The neck should be palpated for cervical lymphadenopathy and extralaryngeal extension. The lesions are visualized with dynamic and rigid laryngoscopy. Vocal cords are assessed for impaired mobility due to tumor burden or anatomic fixation. Computed tomography (CT) and MRI are used complementarily in surgical planning. CT is useful for the evaluation of sclerotic changes or erosion in the case of cartilage or bone involvement. MRI is helpful to

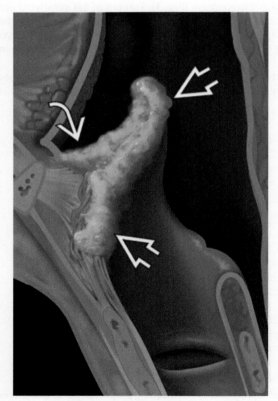

Fig. 2. A suprahyoid laryngeal epiglottic cancer destroying the epiglottic cartilage and hyoepiglottic ligament barrier, facilitating invasion of the preglottic space and vallecula (*curved arrow*), sagittal view. (*From* Gurgel RK, Harnsberger HR. Staging: Larynx. In: Harnsberger HR, ed. Imaging in Otolaryngology. Elsevier; [2018]:240-244.)

demonstrate submucosal or transglottic spread, preepiglottic or paraglottic involvement, as well as tumor invasion into the cartilage.

In CLS, pulmonary function is an important aspect to consider. Patients should be able to tolerate some degree of aspiration postoperatively, as this is likely an inevitable short-term consequence of CLS. As such, patients with severe chronic obstructive pulmonary disorder or emphysema may not be appropriate candidates for laryngeal preservation procedures. Assessment of pulmonary function can be performed with a simple questionnaire about their ability to perform daily activities or with pulmonary function tests. Patients should be consented and prepared for total laryngectomy for potential tumor spread beyond the expected preoperative evaluation. Speech pathology should evaluate patients preoperatively to help identify the right candidates for surgery and for postoperative expectations.

COMPLIANCE WITH GUIDELINES

The American Society of Clinical Oncology updated recommendations on the use of laryngeal preservation strategies in 2018.[18]

a. Early-stage laryngeal cancer: In early stage T1 and T2 laryngeal cancers, patients should be treated with single modality of either radiation or surgery. In cases of verrucous carcinoma resistant to radiation, surgery is favored.
b. Late-stage laryngeal cancer: Patients with T3 and T4 laryngeal cancers are managed with dual modality treatment; surgery with postoperative radiation or concurrent chemoradiation. They can still be a candidate for CLS such as SCPL; however, both patient and physician must be aware of the risk of requiring a future total laryngectomy secondary to tracheostomy dependence and/or aspiration requiring a gastrostomy tube for nutritional support. Patients with a preoperative nonfunctional larynx or cartilage involvement should undergo primary total laryngectomy. Rarely, patients with advanced stage laryngeal cancers may undergo primary radiation therapy with salvage total laryngectomy after if they wish to retain their larynx and are not a candidate for chemotherapy or laryngeal preservation surgery. This yields similar survival to patients who undergo chemoradiation.

TYPES OF CONSERVATION LARYNGEAL SURGERIES
Transoral Endoscopic Resection

Endoscopic microsurgery is the preferred surgical approach to early-stage laryngeal carcinoma. While open approaches afford better exposure, they bear greater morbidity including the need for temporary tracheostomy or feeding tube placement. In a 2009 meta-analysis of 7600 patients who underwent transoral laser microsurgery (TLM) versus radiotherapy for early-stage glottic cancers, there was no difference in local control and laryngectomy-free survival rates. The analysis found that TLM yielded better overall survival, whereas voice outcomes were superior with radiotherapy.[19] For earliest stage cancer (T1a) with a normal or diminished mucosal wave, Schrijvers and colleagues demonstrated that the 5 year laryngeal preservation rate among patients undergoing TLM is superior to the 5 year laryngeal preservation rate of those receiving definitive radiation (95% vs 77%, respectively).[20]

The treatment decision should be based on physician expertise, patient preference, and available resources. Patients with poor laryngeal exposure should not proceed with TLM. It should be noted that, in patients who received primary radiation, surveillance of recurrence may be difficult due to postradiation edema, and vocal fold mobility may be likewise affected by radiation. This leads to delayed detection and more advanced recurrence, which may impede salvage CLS. Only one-third of recurrent early laryngeal cancers after primary radiation are amenable to salvage CLS.[21–23] The risk of a laryngectomy is 12.7 fold higher in patients treated with primary radiation compared to those treated with transoral laser surgery.[21] Also important to note, a second primary cancer is not uncommon among patients with a history of head and neck cancer, and preserving radiation for subsequent head and neck malignancies may be a reasonable choice.

In early laryngeal cancer, the goal of surgical resection is to achieve negative margins while maximizing laryngeal preservation and function. In cases where residual tumor is suspected, re-resection is preferred over adjuvant radiation per current guideline recommendations.[18] The presence of positive margins during the initial resection can negatively impact local control during re-resection. Therefore, disease eradication at the initial resection is emphasized.[24] Endoscopic re-resection in the case of early detection of recurrence demonstrates reasonable local control rates with laser alone (93.4%, 95%, and 85.6% for Tis, T1, and T2, respectively).[25] In patients with minimal invasion of lamina propria, vocal stripping and deep excision are avoided, whereas photoablation with preservation of most of lamina propria will maintain vocal cord pliability. A cautious approach is warranted for cancer with deep vocal cord invasion or involving the anterior commissure. Surgical exposure should be considered, and resection to negative margins may create a large defect with resultant dysphonia and aspiration risk. T2b glottic cancer with impaired vocal mobility may signal extraconal involvement and open laryngeal surgery may thus be considered.

In early supraglottic cancer, avoidance of multimodal treatment is similarly prioritized. Surgical treatment of supraglottic cancer typically requires bilateral neck dissection and, accordingly, a combination of neck dissection and endoscopic surgery or open laryngeal surgery may be pursued. Canis and colleagues illustrated a 2 year local control rate of 93% for T1/2 supraglottic cancer treated with TLM.[26] Iro and colleagues demonstrated a 5 year local control of 85.0% for T1 and 62.6% for T2 supraglottic tumors with TLM.[27] Endoscopic resection of supraglottic cancer has yielded similar outcomes to open laryngeal surgery or radiation in terms of locoregional control and overall survival.[28] In the setting of frequent second primary and recurrence in these patients with laryngeal cancer, primary surgery may be a preferred approach.

TLM has also been used for late-stage laryngeal cancers in some cases. Perreti and colleagues found that the 5 year local control rate was 71.6% and the laryngeal preservation rate was 72.7% for patients with T3 glottic squamous cell carcinoma (SCC) treated with TLM.[29] The lateral and posterior paraglottic space should be closely attended to. Suboptimal control in these areas may lead to recurrence. Wider resection with the removal of perichondrium of thyroid lamina or piecemeal removal to ensure complete clearance of cancer can be done.[29] The frequency of significant surgical and medical complications is less than what is typically reported following open partial laryngectomies and nonsurgical organ preservation protocols.[30] Functional preservation is superior for T3 supraglottic tumors compared to glottic.[31]

Open conservation laryngeal surgeries

With the advent of TLM, the role of open CLS has declined significantly for early laryngeal cancer.[31] In the following discussions, we delineate various open CLS procedures and their respective applications.

Vertical partial laryngectomy. This procedure was designed to resect glottic cancer with partial removal of the thyroid cartilage and paraglottic space. It is considered obsolete in the advent of TLM and radiation. The local control rate is excellent with this technique for T1 glottic carcinoma. Desanto and colleagues published their series of 211 patients with vertical partial laryngectomy (VPL) for T1 glottic cancer; only 10 patients developed recurrence at the 5 year follow-up.[32] Another sizable study echoed these favorable outcomes, reporting a remarkable local control rate of 93% for T1 glottic cancer; however, they cautioned the need to take wide margins at the anterior commissure to prevent subglottic recurrence.[33] Indications for this procedure include glottic cancers with superficial spread spanning from the vocal process to the contra-lateral anterior one-third of the vocal cord. Caution is warranted when impaired mobility suggests potential extension of glottic cancer into the paraglottic space, with a heightened incidence of local failure in patients with T2 and T3 glottic carcinoma across various series.[33–36] Hoarseness is the predominant adverse laryngeal outcome.[37] Postoperatively, the rates of aspiration pneumonia and permanent trache-ostomy are less than 2%, underscoring the rehabilitative success of this procedure.[36]

Horizontal partial laryngectomy

Supraglottic laryngectomy This procedure is typically employed for managing T1 and T2 supraglottic carcinomas, especially when endoscopic resection is not possible. It involves the resection of a substantial portion of the thyroid cartilage, while judiciously preserving the lower segment of the thyroid cartilage as well as the aryte-noids and true cords. Several studies reported local recurrence rates of 0% to 10% for T1 and 0% to 15% for T2 supraglottic cancers.[38–40] The oncologic outcome improved with the use of adjuvant radiation in higher stage supraglottic cancer.[39,41] Decannula-tion was achieved in 96% of cases, and nasogastric tube removal was achieved in 84% of the patients within 30 days.[40] Herranz-Gonzalez and colleagues advised reducing all tissues from the supraglottis and not to reconstruct with mucosal flap over the arytenoid to facilitate decannulation.[40] Phonation is generally preserved with conservation of both vocal cords. Up to 67% of patients experience only mild dysphonia or no significant voice changes after postsupraglottic laryngectomy.[42] This procedure should not be used when tumors extend to either arytenoid or the glottis. Once the tumor penetrates the thyroid cartilage, it is difficult to predict if the spared lower thyroid cartilage is uninvolved. Therefore, thyroid cartilage invasion is likewise a contraindication to supraglottic laryngectomy.

Supracricoid partial laryngectomy This procedure resects the thyroid cartilage en bloc with the paraglottic space, bilateral false cords, and true cords. At least one cri-coarytenoid unit should be preserved. SCPL has regained popularity due to the ability to treat high-stage tumors while still conserving laryngeal function as an alternative to total laryngectomy. SCPL is contraindicated in patients with significant involvement of the preepiglottic space or the hyoid.

a. Glottic carcinoma: Primary candidates for this procedure include patients with un-favorable T2, T3, and select T4 glottic carcinomas. SCPL facilitates removal of higher stage tumors than VPL due to complete resection of thyroid cartilage and paraglottic space. A superior 10 year local control rate for T2 glottic cancer was observed with SCPL at 94.6% compared to 69.3% with VPL.[33] Cases with thyroid cartilage invasion are amenable to this procedure and result in similar oncologic outcomes to total laryngectomy. Laudadio and colleagues found that the 5 year actuarial disease-free survival was 85% in 206 patients with T1–T4 laryngeal carci-nomas who underwent SCPL.[43] The functional organ preservation rate was high, at 97%, with normal swallowing in 93.7% of the patients by the end of the first post-operative month.[43] Beyond primary cancer resection, SCPL offers a valuable salvage option for patients with recurrence following primary radiotherapy or more conservative procedures such as VPL or TLM. This multifaceted utility positions SCPL as a versatile and effective tool in the management of advanced laryngeal carcinomas.[43,44]

b. Supraglottic carcinoma: SCPL may be employed for more advanced supraglottic tumors than supraglottic laryngectomy, as it allows for the removal of at least one cricoarytenoid unit and complete resection of the thyroid cartilage. Laccourreye and colleagues published outcomes of a series of 68 patients who received SCPL primarily with T2 and T3 supraglottic cancers. The 3 year overall survival rate reached 71.4% with no identifiable local recurrence.[45] Most available series around the world adopting this procedure for T2 and T3 supraglottic cancers report local recurrence rates in the single digits from 0% to 9%.[45–49]

The functional outcomes after SCPL vary and are dependent on surgeons' experience and treatment with adjuvant radiation. Lewin and colleagues reported that all patients in their cohort experienced aspiration due to neoglottic incompetency, alongside impaired base of tongue and laryngeal movements. Postoperatively, more than half the patients needed temporary gastrostomy tubes, but 81% of patients returned to complete oral intake.[50] The authors advocate for meticulous patient selection encompassing thorough preoperative assessments of pulmonary and swallow function, and the patient's ability to participate in postoperative dysphagia rehabilitation. Other studies have found the ultimate need for functional total laryngectomy is low, less than 5%.[51–53] Risk factors for dysphagia include increased age, arytenoid resection, failure to resuspend the piriform sinus anteriorly, epiglottis removal, and hypoglossal nerve injury.

Transoral Robotic Surgery

Despite its established role in oropharyngeal cancer treatment, the utilization of transoral robotic surgery (TORS) in laryngeal cancer is currently limited and subject to ongoing investigation. TORS offers an expansive field of exposure with magnification and ergonomic manipulation of instruments, allowing surgeons to rest their hands or wrists comfortably at the console. Transoral robotic supraglottic laryngectomy stands out as the primary application of TORS in laryngeal cancer and is typically employed for early T1–T2 and some T3 tumors. In a multicenter observational study of 122 patients in France, the local control rate following TORS for early-stage or intermediate-stage supraglottic cancer was at least comparable to open or transoral laser surgery.[54] TORS has also been used for cordectomy and advocated for use in tumors involving the anterior commissure for which TLM exposure is difficult.[55]

Due to the scarcity and heterogeneity of literature on TORS for laryngeal cancer, reports on the complication rate are not reliable and depend on the surgeon's technical skills and patient selection. Rates of definitive percutaneous gastrostomy and tracheostomy after TORS supraglottic laryngectomy at 9.5% and 1%, respectively.[56] The same study reported rates of aspiration pneumonia and postoperative bleeding requiring reoperation at 23% and 14%, respectively.[56] Others report a lower bleeding rate (3.74% in 503 patients), commonly managed by ligation of the internal branch of the superior laryngeal artery.[57] Further studies are required to clearly define the indications and contraindications to TORS in the management of laryngeal cancer and to outline postoperative complications in order to better guide surgical decision-making.

NONSURGICAL OPTIONS

The pivotal trials conducted by the Department of Veterans Affairs (VA) Laryngeal Cancer Study Group and the Intergroup Radiation Therapy Oncology Group (RTOG 91–11) have significantly shaped the landscape of treatment recommendations for late-stage laryngeal cancer. The consensus arising from these trials supports chemoradiation for T3 and selected T4a cancers, aiming to circumvent total laryngectomy to preserve laryngeal function.[58,59]

Dziegielewski and colleagues' comparative analysis of T3 and T4a laryngeal cancers in Canada revealed intriguing insights; the 5 year survival rate for total laryngectomy with adjuvant radiation versus primary chemoradiation were 70% versus 52% for T3 cancers and 49% versus 16% for T4a cancers, respectively.[60] Moreover, a National Cancer Database analysis found upfront total laryngectomy is superior to primary chemoradiation for T4 laryngeal cancer, HR of 1.55.[61] MD Anderson Cancer Center's investigation echoed these results, affirming better locoregional control achieved with total laryngectomy and adjuvant radiation, but ultimately, a comparable overall median survival was observed between the 2 approaches.[62] Regarding laryngeal function outcomes, 45% of the laryngeal preservation patients had a posttreatment tracheostomy, and the rate of tube feed dependence was higher in the larynx preservation group compared to total laryngectomy and adjuvant radiation group (17% vs 7%, respectively).[62]

In the VA trial, salvage laryngectomy was required in up to 56% of T4a cancers.[58] The high salvage laryngectomy rate after chemoradiation may be due to poor patient selection. Accordingly, a comprehensive assessment of a patient's airway and swallowing function is imperative in guiding treatment decisions. Individuals exhibiting compromised laryngeal function marked by aspiration, severe dysphagia, or tracheostomy dependence should undergo total laryngectomy coupled with adjuvant radiation. Patients with advanced laryngeal cancer and thyroid cartilage involvement also demonstrate impaired laryngeal incompetence after radiation or chemoradiation; thus, total laryngectomy or SCPL is recommended.

As outlined earlier, SCPL can be effective for laryngeal preservation in T3 and some T4a cancers. Lima and colleagues performed SCPL-CHEP in 43 advanced glottic cancers T3 and T4; only 6.9% had local recurrences at 5 years, and 74.4% of patients attained normal swallowing.[63] Weinstein and colleagues studied whole organ sections of total laryngectomy specimens and found that many patients may have been candidates for SCPL.[64]

SUMMARY

This review is intended to guide surgeons in their management of laryngeal cancer. For early-stage tumors, single modality treatment with radiation or surgery is preferred. While radiation may yield more favorable voice outcomes, the challenge lies in its potential to impede the detection of recurrence. Primary radiation may likewise restrict management options in the setting of recurrence, and salvage surgery postradiation can be complicated by the inability to distinguish between cancer and postradiation changes. For late-stage cancer, combined treatments of surgery with adjuvant radiation/chemoradiation or concurrent chemoradiation are standards of care. Management selection should be guided by the pretreatment assessment of laryngeal function and medical comorbidities. Patients with tracheostomy tube dependence and severe dysphagia are better treated with total laryngectomy followed by adjuvant radiation. Supracricoid laryngectomy offers a valuable alternative to total laryngectomy in select cases including salvage resection. Surgeon experience and comfort with the surgical approaches to larynx cancer strongly influence functional and oncologic outcomes, and accordingly surgeons must establish a deep understanding of indications and risks associated with each procedure.

CLINICS CARE POINTS

- For the treatment of early laryngeal cancer, a preferred approach involves a single modality, either radiation or surgery, with superior voice outcomes associated with radiation.
- In cases of late-stage cancer, the current recommendation is a combination of treatments, such as surgery with adjuvant radiation/chemoradiation or concurrent chemoradiation. Total laryngectomy followed by postoperative radiation is strongly considered for patients with tracheostomy tube dependence, severe dysphagia, and thyroid cartilage penetration.

DISCLOSURE

The authors have nothing to disclose.

REFERENCES

1. National Cancer Institute, Surveillance, Epidemiology, and End Results Program. "Cancer Stat Facts: Larynx Cancer." SEER Cancer Statistics. Available at: https://seer.cancer.gov/statfacts/html/laryn.html.
2. Hashibe M, Brennan P, Chuang S-C, et al. Interaction between tobacco and alcohol use and the risk of head and neck cancer: pooled analysis in the International Head and Neck Cancer Epidemiology Consortium. Cancer Epidemiol Biomarkers Prev 2009;18(2):541–50.
3. Gama RR, Carvalho AL, Filho AL, et al. Detection of human papillomavirus in laryngeal squamous cell carcinoma: systematic review and meta-analysis. Laryngoscope 2016;126(4):885–93.
4. Ndiaye C, Mena M, Alemany L, et al. HPV DNA, E6/E7 mRNA, and p16INK4a detection in head and neck cancers: a systematic review and meta-analysis. Lancet Oncol 2014;15(13):1319–31.
5. Groome PA, O'Sullivan B, Irish JC, et al. Management and outcome differences in supraglottic cancer between Ontario, Canada, and the Surveillance, Epidemiology, and End Results areas of the United States. J Clin Oncol 2003;21(3): 496–505.
6. Bosetti C, Gallus S, Franceschi S, et al. Cancer of the larynx in non-smoking alcohol drinkers and in non-drinking tobacco smokers. Br J Cancer 2002;87(5): 516–8.
7. Schwartz AW. Dr. Theodor Billroth and the first laryngectomy. Ann Plast Surg 1978;1(5):513–6.
8. Kirchner JA, Carter D. Intralaryngeal barriers to the spread of cancer. Acta Otolaryngol 1987;103(5–6):503–13.
9. Kirchner JA, Baker DC Jr. Memorial lecture. What have whole organ sections contributed to the treatment of laryngeal cancer? Ann Otol Rhinol Laryngol 1989;98(9):661–7. PMID: 2782798.
10. Bagatella F, Bignardi L. Morphological study of the laryngeal anterior commissure with regard to the spread of cancer. Acta Otolaryngol 1981;92(1–2):167–71.
11. Ulusan M, Unsaler S, Basaran B, et al. The incidence of thyroid cartilage invasion through the anterior commissure in clinically early-staged laryngeal cancer. Eur Arch Oto-Rhino-Laryngol 2016;273:447–53.
12. Kirchner JA, Som ML. Clinical and histological observations on supraglottic cancer. Ann Otol Rhinol Laryngol 1971;80:638–44.

13. Leroux-Robert J. Statistical study of 620 laryngeal carcinoma of the glottic region personally operated on more than 5 years ago (1955-1969) [in French]. Ann Otolaryngol Chir Cervicofac 1974;91(9):445–58.
14. Nakayama M, Brandenburg JH. Clinical Underestimation of Laryngeal Cancer: Predictive Indicators. Arch Otolaryngol Head Neck Surg 1993;119(9):950–7.
15. Timon CI, Gullane PJ, Brown D, et al. Hyoid bone involvement by squamous cell carcinoma: clinical and pathological features. Laryngoscope 1992;102(5): 515–20. PMID: 1573947.
16. Petrović Z, Krejović B, Djukić V, et al. Primary surgical treatment for carcinoma of the larynx: influence of the local invasion. J Laryngol Otol 1991;105(5):353–5. PMID: 2040837.
17. Zeitels SM, Vaughan CW. Preepiglottic space invasion in "early" epiglottic cancer. Ann Otol Rhinol Laryngol 1991;100(10):789–92.
18. Forastiere AA, Ismaila N, Lewin JS, et al. Use of Larynx-Preservation Strategies in the Treatment of Laryngeal Cancer: American Society of Clinical Oncology Clinical Practice Guideline Update. J Clin Oncol 2018;36(11):1143–69. Epub 2017 Nov 27. PMID: 29172863.
19. Higgins KM, Shah MD, Ogaick MJ, et al. Treatment of early-stage glottic cancer: meta-analysis comparison of laser excision versus radiotherapy. J Otolaryngol Head Neck Surg 2009;38(6):603–12. PMID: 19958721.
20. Schrijvers ML, van Riel EL, Langendijk JA, et al. Higher laryngeal preservation rate after CO_2 laser surgery compared with radiotherapy in T1a glottic laryngeal carcinoma. Head Neck 2009;31(6):759–64.
21. Warner L, Lee K, Homer JJ. Transoral laser microsurgery versus radiotherapy for T2 glottic squamous cell carcinoma: a systematic review of local control outcomes. Clin Otolaryngol 2017;42(3):629–36.
22. Desanto LW, Lillie JC, Devine KD. Surgical salvage after radiation for laryngeal cancer. Laryngoscope 1976;86:649–57.
23. McLaughlin MP, Parsons JT, Fein DA, et al. Salvage surgery after radiotherapy failure in T1–T2 squamous cell carcinoma of the glottic larynx. Head Neck 1996;18:229–35.
24. Ganly I, Patel SG, Matsuo J, et al. Results of surgical salvage after failure of definitive radiation therapy for early-stage squamous cell carcinoma of the glottic larynx. Arch Otolaryngol Head Neck Surg 2006;132:59–66.
25. Jäckel MC, Ambrosch P, Martin A, et al. Impact of re-resection for inadequate margins on the prognosis of upper aerodigestive tract cancer treated by laser microsurgery. Laryngoscope 2007;117:350–6.
26. Canis M, Martin A, Ihler F, et al. Results of transoral laser microsurgery for supraglottic carcinoma in 277 patients. Eur Arch Oto-Rhino-Laryngol 2013;270(8): 2315–26. Epub 2013 Jan 10. PMID: 23306348; PMCID: PMC3699705.
27. Iro H, Waldfahrer F, Altendorf-Hofmann A, et al. Transoral Laser Surgery of Supraglottic Cancer: Follow-up of 141 Patients. Arch Otolaryngol Head Neck Surg 1998;124(11):1245–50.
28. Bumber Z, Prgomet D, Janjanin S. Endoscopic CO_2 laser surgery for supraglottic cancer–ten years of experience. Coll Antropol 2009;33:87–91.
29. Peretti G, Piazza C, Penco S, et al. Transoral laser microsurgery as primary treatment for selected T3 glottic and supraglottic cancers. Head Neck 2016;38: 1107–12.
30. Vilaseca I, Blanch JL, Berenguer J, et al. Transoral laser microsurgery for locally advanced (T3-T4a) supraglottic squamous cell carcinoma: sixteen years of experience. Head Neck 2016;38:1050–7.

31. Silver CE, Beitler JJ, Shaha AR, et al. Current trends in the initial management of laryngeal cancer: the declining use of open surgery. Eur Arch Oto-Rhino-Laryngol 2009;266(9):1333–52. Epub 2009 Jul 14. PMID: 19597837.

32. DeSanto LW. Cancer of the larynx–Mayo Clinic experience 1970-1980. Rochester, MN: Presented at the Mayo Clinic Alumni Meeting; 1983.

33. Laccourreye O, Weinstein G, Brasnu D, et al. Vertical partial laryngectomy: a critical analysis of local recurrence. Ann Otol Rhinol Laryngol 1991;100:68.

34. Kirchner J, Som ML. The anterior commissure technique of partial laryngectomy: clinical and laboratory observations. Laryngoscope 1975;85:1308.

35. Biller HF, Lawson W. Partial laryngectomy for vocal cord cancer with marked limitation or fixation of the vocal cord. Laryngoscope 1986;96:61.

36. Laccourreye O, Laccourreye L, Garcia D, et al. Vertical partial laryngectomy versus supracricoid partial laryngectomy for selected carcinomas of the true vocal cord classified as T2N0. Ann Otol Rhinol Laryngol 2000;109:965–71.

37. Hirano M, Kurita S, Matsuoka H. Vocal function following hemilaryngectomy. Ann Otol Rhinol Laryngol 1987;96:586.

38. Bocca E, Pignataro O, Oldini C, et al. Extended supraglottic laryngectomy. Review of 84 cases. Ann Otol Rhinol Laryngol 1987;96:384.

39. Burstein FD, Calcaterra TC. Supraglottic laryngectomy: series report and analysis of results. Laryngoscope 1985;95:833.

40. Herranz-González J, Gavilán J, Martínez-Vidal J, et al. Supraglottic laryngectomy: functional and oncologic results. Ann Otol Rhinol Laryngol 1996;105:18.

41. Robbins KT, Davidson W, Peters LJ, et al. Conservation Surgery for T2 and T3 Carcinomas of the Supraglottic Larynx. Arch Otolaryngol Head Neck Surg 1988;114(4):421–6.

42. Klein AD, Wasserstrom JP, Sessions DG, et al. Rehabilitation of partial laryngectomy patients. Trans Am Acad Ophthalmol Otolaryngol 1977;84:324.

43. Laudadio P, Presutti L, Dall'Olio D, et al. Supracricoid laryngectomies: Long-term oncological and functional results. Acta Otolaryngol 2006;126(6):640–9.

44. Weinstein GS, El-Sawy MM, Ruiz C, et al. Laryngeal preservation with supracricoid partial laryngectomy results in improved quality of life when compared with total laryngectomy. Laryngoscope 2001;111(2):191–9.

45. Laccourreye H, Laccourreye O, Weinstein G, et al. Supracricoid laryngectomy with cricohyoidopexy: A partial laryngeal procedure for selected supraglottic and transglottic carcinomas. Laryngoscope 1990;100:735–41.

46. Chevalier D, Piquet JJ. Subtotal laryngectomy with cricohyoidopexy for supraglottic carcinoma: review of 61 cases. Am J Surg 1994;168:472.

47. Schwaab G, Kolb F, Julieron M, et al. Subtotal laryngectomy with cricohyoidopexy as first treatment procedure for supraglottic carcinoma: institut Gustave-Roussy experience (146 cases, 1974-1997). Eur Arch Oto-Rhino-Laryngol 2001;258:246–9.

48. Karasalihoglu AR, Yagiz R, Tas A, et al. Supracricoid partial laryngectomy with cricohyoidopexy and cricohyoidoepiglottopexy: functional and oncological results. J Laryngol Otol 2004;118:671–5.

49. Souldi H, Rouadi S, Abada R, et al. Clinical outcome of supracricoid partial laryngectomy: experience on 31 patients. J Surg 2017;5:1–4.

50. Lewin JS, Hutcheson KA, Barringer DA, et al. Functional analysis of swallowing outcomes after supracricoid partial laryngectomy. Head Neck 2008;30(5):559–66.

51. Guerrier B, Lallemant JG, Balmigere G, et al. Our experience in reconstructive surgery in glottic cancers. Ann Otolaryngol Chir Cervicofac 1987;104:175.

52. Pech A, Cannoni M, Giovanni A, et al. Requisite selection of surgical technics in the treatment of cancer of the larynx. Ann Otolaryngol Chir Cervicofac 1986; 103:565.

53. Naudo P, Laccourreye O, Weinstein G, et al. Complications and functional outcome after supracricoid partial laryngectomy with cricohyoidoepiglottopexy. Otolaryngol Head Neck Surg 1998;118:124–9.

54. Doazan M, Hans S, Morinière S, et al. Oncologic outcomes with transoral robotic surgery for supraglottic squamous cell carcinoma: Results of the French Robotic Surgery Group of GETTEC. Head Neck 2018;40(9):2050–9.

55. Wang CC, Lin WJ, Wang JJ, et al. Transoral Robotic Surgery for Early-T Stage Glottic Cancer Involving the Anterior Commissure-News and Update. Front Oncol 2022;12:755400.

56. Razafindranaly V, Lallemant B, Aubry K, et al. Clinical outcomes with transoral robotic surgery for supraglottic squamous cell carcinoma: Experience of a French evaluation cooperative subgroup of GETTEC. Head Neck 2016;38:E1097–101.

57. Turner MT, Stokes WA, Stokes CM, et al. Airway and bleeding complications of transoral robotic supraglottic laryngectomy (TORS-SGL): A systematic review and meta-analysis. Oral Oncol 2021;118:105301.

58. Department of Veterans Affairs Laryngeal Cancer Study Group, Wolf GT, Fisher SG, Hong WK, et al. Induction chemotherapy plus radiation compared with surgery plus radiation in patients with advanced laryngeal cancer. N Engl J Med 1991;324(24):1685–90. PMID: 2034244.

59. Forastiere AA, Zhang Q, Weber RS, et al. Long-term results of RTOG 91-11: a comparison of three nonsurgical treatment strategies to preserve the larynx in patients with locally advanced larynx cancer. J Clin Oncol 2013;31(7):845–52.

60. Dziegielewski PT, O'Connell DA, Klein M, et al. Primary total laryngectomy versus organ preservation for T3/T4a laryngeal cancer: a population-based analysis of survival. J Otolaryngol Head Neck Surg 2012;41(Suppl 1):S56–64. PMID: 22569051.

61. Stokes WA, Jones BL, Bhatia S, et al. A comparison of overall survival for patients with T4 larynx cancer treated with surgical versus organ-preservation approaches: A National Cancer Data Base analysis. Cancer 2017;123(4):600–8.

62. Rosenthal DI, Mohamed ASR, Weber RS, et al. Long-term outcomes after surgical or nonsurgical initial therapy for patients with T4 squamous cell carcinoma of the larynx: A 3-decade survey. Cancer 2015;121:1608–19.

63. Lima RA, Freitas EQ, Dias FL, et al. Supracricoid laryngectomy with cricohyoidoepiglottopexy for advanced glottic cancer. Head Neck 2006;28:481–6.

64. Weinstein GS, El-Sawy MM, Ruiz C, et al. Laryngeal Preservation With Supracricoid Partial Laryngectomy Results in Improved Quality of Life When Compared With Total Laryngectomy. Laryngoscope 2001;111:191–9.

UNITED STATES POSTAL SERVICE ®

Statement of Ownership, Management, and Circulation
(All Periodicals Publications Except Requester Publications)

1. Publication Title	2. Publication Number	3. Filing Date
SURGICAL ONCOLOGY CLINICS OF NORTH AMERICA	012 – 565	9/18/2024

4. Issue Frequency	5. Number of Issues Published Annually	6. Annual Subscription Price
JAN, APR, JUL, OCT	4	$345.00

7. Complete Mailing Address of Known Office of Publication (Not printer) (Street, city, county, state, and ZIP+4®)

ELSEVIER INC.
230 Park Avenue, Suite 800
New York, NY 10169

Contact Person
Malathi Samayan

Telephone (Include area code)
91-44-4299-4507

8. Complete Mailing Address of Headquarters or General Business Office of Publisher (Not printer)

ELSEVIER INC.
230 Park Avenue, Suite 800
New York, NY 10169

9. Full Names and Complete Mailing Addresses of Publisher, Editor, and Managing Editor (Do not leave blank)

Publisher (Name and complete mailing address)

Dolores Meloni, ELSEVIER INC.
1600 JOHN F KENNEDY BLVD. SUITE 1600
PHILADELPHIA, PA 19103-2899

Editor (Name and complete mailing address)

JOHN VASSALLO, ELSEVIER INC.
1600 JOHN F KENNEDY BLVD. SUITE 1600
PHILADELPHIA, PA 19103-2899

Managing Editor (Name and complete mailing address)

PATRICK MANLEY, ELSEVIER INC.
1600 JOHN F KENNEDY BLVD. SUITE 1600
PHILADELPHIA, PA 19103-2899

10. Owner (Do not leave blank. If the publication is owned by a corporation, give the name and address of the corporation immediately followed by the names and addresses of all stockholders owning or holding 1 percent or more of the total amount of stock. If not owned by a corporation, give the names and addresses of the individual owners. If owned by a partnership or other unincorporated firm, give its name and address as well as those of each individual owner. If the publication is published by a nonprofit organization, give its name and address.)

Full Name	Complete Mailing Address
WHOLLY OWNED SUBSIDIARY OF REED/ELSEVIER, US HOLDINGS	1600 JOHN F KENNEDY BLVD. SUITE 1600 PHILADELPHIA, PA 19103-2899

11. Known Bondholders, Mortgagees, and Other Security Holders Owning or Holding 1 Percent or More of Total Amount of Bonds, Mortgages, or Other Securities. If none, check box. ► ☐ None

Full Name	Complete Mailing Address
N/A	

12. Tax Status (For completion by nonprofit organizations authorized to mail at nonprofit rates) (Check one)

The purpose, function, and nonprofit status of this organization and the exempt status for federal income tax purposes:

☒ Has Not Changed During Preceding 12 Months
☐ Has Changed During Preceding 12 Months (Publisher must submit explanation of change with this statement)

PS Form **3526**, July 2014 [Page 1 of 4 (see instructions page 4)] PSN: 7530-01-000-9931 PRIVACY NOTICE: See our privacy policy on www.usps.com.

---

13. Publication Title	14. Issue Date for Circulation Data Below
SURGICAL ONCOLOGY CLINICS OF NORTH AMERICA	JULY 2024

15. Extent and Nature of Circulation		Average No. Copies Each Issue During Preceding 12 Months	No. Copies of Single Issue Published Nearest to Filing Date
a. Total Number of Copies (Net press run)		82	77
b. Paid Circulation (By Mail and Outside the Mail)	(1) Mailed Outside-County Paid Subscriptions Stated on PS Form 3541 (Include paid distribution above nominal rate, advertiser's proof copies, and exchange copies)	50	42
	(2) Mailed In-County Paid Subscriptions Stated on PS Form 3541 (Include paid distribution above nominal rate, advertiser's proof copies, and exchange copies)	0	0
	(3) Paid Distribution Outside the Mails Including Sales Through Dealers and Carriers, Street Vendors, Counter Sales, and Other Paid Distribution Outside USPS®	19	18
	(4) Paid Distribution by Other Classes of Mail Through the USPS (e.g., First-Class Mail®)	13	17
c. Total Paid Distribution (Sum of 15b (1), (2), (3), and (4))	►	82	77
d. Free or Nominal Rate Distribution (By Mail and Outside the Mail)	(1) Free or Nominal Rate Outside-County Copies Included on PS Form 3541	0	0
	(2) Free or Nominal Rate In-County Copies Included on PS Form 3541	0	0
	(3) Free or Nominal Rate Copies Mailed at Other Classes Through the USPS (e.g., First-Class Mail)	0	0
	(4) Free or Nominal Rate Distribution Outside the Mail (Carriers or other means)	0	0
e. Total Free or Nominal Rate Distribution (Sum of 15d (1), (2), (3) and (4))	►	0	0
f. Total Distribution (Sum of 15c and 15e)	►	82	77
g. Copies not Distributed (See Instructions to Publishers #4 (page 3))	►	0	0
h. Total (Sum of 15f and g)	►	82	77
i. Percent Paid (15c divided by 15f times 100)	►	100%	100%

* If you are claiming electronic copies, go to line 16 on page 3. If you are not claiming electronic copies, skip to line 17 on page 3.

16. Electronic Copy Circulation	Average No. Copies Each Issue During Preceding 12 Months	No. Copies of Single Issue Published Nearest to Filing Date
a. Paid Electronic Copies	►	
b. Total Paid Print Copies (Line 15c) + Paid Electronic Copies (Line 16a)	►	
c. Total Print Distribution (Line 15f) + Paid Electronic Copies (Line 16a)	►	
d. Percent Paid (Both Print & Electronic Copies) (16b divided by 16c × 100)	►	

☒ I certify that 50% of all my distributed copies (electronic and print) are paid above a nominal price.

17. Publication of Statement of Ownership

☒ If the publication is a general publication, publication of this statement is required. Will be printed in the **OCTOBER 2024** issue of this publication.

☐ Publication not required.

18. Signature and Title of Editor, Publisher, Business Manager, or Owner		Date
Malathi Samayan - Distribution Controller	*Malathi Samayan*	9/18/2024

I certify that all information furnished on this form is true and complete. I understand that anyone who furnishes false or misleading information on this form or who omits material or information requested on the form may be subject to criminal sanctions (including fines and imprisonment) and/or civil sanctions (including civil penalties).

PS Form **3526**, July 2014 (Page 3 of 4) PRIVACY NOTICE: See our privacy policy on www.usps.com

Moving?

Make sure your subscription moves with you!

To notify us of your new address, find your **Clinics Account Number** (located on your mailing label above your name), and contact customer service at:

Email: journalscustomerservice-usa@elsevier.com

800-654-2452 (subscribers in the U.S. & Canada)
314-447-8871 (subscribers outside of the U.S. & Canada)

Fax number: 314-447-8029

Elsevier Health Sciences Division
Subscription Customer Service
3251 Riverport Lane
Maryland Heights, MO 63043